ABC OF BREAST DISEA

Third Edition

Edited by

J MICHAEL DIXON

Consultant surgeon and senior lecturer in surgery, Edinburgh Breast Unit,
Western General Hospital, Edinburgh

BMJ
Books

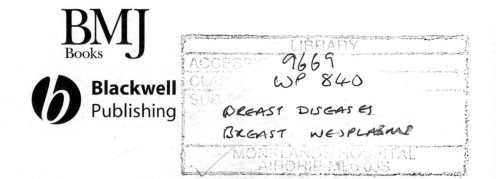

Blackwell
Publishing

© 1995, 2000 BMJ Books
© 2006 by Blackwell Publishing Ltd
BMJ Books is an imprint of the BMJ Publishing Group Limited, used under licence

Blackwell Publishing, Inc., 350 Main Street, Malden, Massachusetts 02148-5020, USA
Blackwell Publishing Ltd, 9600 Garsington Road, Oxford OX4 2DQ, UK
Blackwell Publishing Asia Pty Ltd, 550 Swanston Street, Carlton, Victoria 3053, Australia

First published 1995
Second edition 2000
Third edition 2006

Library of Congress Cataloging-in-Publication Data
ABC of breast diseases/edited by J. Michael Dixon.—3rd ed.
         p.   ;   cm.
     Includes bibliographical references and index.
     ISBN-13: 978-0-7279-1828-4
     ISBN-10: 0-7279-1828-1
     1. Breast—Diseases—Treatment.   2. Breast—Cancer—Treatment.   I. Dixon, J. M. (J. Michael)
     [DNLM: 1. Breast Diseases.   2. Breast Neoplasms.   WP 840   A134 2006]
  RG491A232 2006
  616.99′449—dc22

                                                                        2005020705

ISBN-13: 978 0 7279 1828 4
ISBN-10: 0 7279 1828 1

A catalogue record for this title is available from the British Library

The cover shows a coloured mammogram of an abscess of the areola of a woman's breast seen from
the side. With permission from CRNI/Science Photo Library

Set in 9/11 pt New Baskerville by Newgen Imaging Systems (P) Ltd, Chennai, India
Printed and bound in India by Replika Press Pvt. Ltd, Harayana

Commissioning Editor: Eleanor Lines
Development Editors: Sally Carter, Nick Morgan
Production Controller: Debbie Wyer

For further information on Blackwell Publishing, visit our website:
http://www.blackwellpublishing.com

The publisher's policy is to use permanent paper from mills that operate a sustainable forestry policy,
and which has been manufactured from pulp processed using acid-free and elementary chlorine-free
practices. Furthermore, the publisher ensures that the text paper and cover board used have met
acceptable environmental accreditation standards.

Contents

Contributors

NJ Bundred
Professor of surgical oncology, department of surgery, South Manchester University Hospital, Manchester

S Chua
Oncology research fellow, Royal Marsden Hospital, London

JM Dixon
Consultant surgeon and senior lecturer in surgery, Edinburgh Breast Unit, Western General Hospital, Edinburgh

P Hopwood
Consultant and honorary senior lecturer in psychiatry and psycho-oncology, Christie Hospital NHS Trust, Manchester

J Iddon
Specialist registrar, North West Region, University Hospital of South Manchester

RCF Leonard
Professor of medical oncology, South West Wales Cancer Institute, Singleton Hospital, Swansea

RD Macmillan
Consultant surgeon, Nottingham Breast Institute, Nottingham City Hospital, Nottingham

P Maguire
Professor of Psychiatric Oncology, Cancer Research UK Psychological Medicine Group, Christie Hospital NHS Trust, Manchester

K McPherson
Visiting professor of public health epidemiology, Nuffield Department of Obstetrics and Gynaecology Research Institute, Churchill Hospital, Oxford

DL Page
Professor in the department of pathology, Vanderbilt University Medical Center, Nashville, Tennessee, USA

J Patnick
Director of NHS Cancer Screening Programmes, The Manor House, Sheffield

SE Pinder
Consultant breast pathologist, department of histopathology, Addenbrooke's NHS Trust, Cambridge

A Rodger
Medical director, Beatson Oncology Centre, Western Infirmary, Glasgow

GM Ross
Consultant clinical oncologist, Royal Marsden Hospital, London

JRC Sainsbury
Senior lecturer in surgery, Royal Free and University College Medical School, University College London

IE Smith
Professor of cancer medicine, Royal Marsden Hospital, London

CM Steel
Professor in medical science, University of St Andrew's, Bute Medical School, St Andrew's, Fife

J Thomas
Consultant pathologist, Western General Hospital, Edinburgh

AM Thompson
Professor of surgical oncology and honorary consultant surgeon, Ninewells Hospital and Medical School, University of Dundee, Dundee

JD Watson
Consultant plastic surgeon, St John's Hospital at Howden, West Lothian

EM Weiler-Mithoff
Consultant plastic and reconstructive surgeon, Canniesburn unit, Glasgow Royal Infirmary, Glasgow

ARM Wilson
Clinical director, Nottingham Breast Institute, Nottingham City Hospital, Nottingham

JR Yarnold
Consultant clinical oncologist, Royal Marsden NHS Trust, Surrey

Preface

The aim of the third edition of the *ABC of Breast Diseases* is to provide an up to date, concise, well illustrated, and evidence based text that will meet the dual challenges of managing the increasing numbers of women who attend breast clinics and the increasing numbers of women who are diagnosed with breast cancer. This edition contains many new illustrations and diagrams. The chapters on screening, adjuvant therapy, clinical trials, and prognostic factors have been completely rewritten, and all other chapters have been extensively revised. The topics of adjuvant therapy and metastatic breast cancer have been extended to cover the explosion of results gained from the many multinational breast cancer trials which have reported since the last edition of this ABC was published. New authors have added their work to that of those who have already contributed to the success of the book. Thanks to Jan Mauritzen my PA who has coordinated the many revisions, to Eleanor Lines. Commissioning Editor, ABC series, to Sally Carter, Development Editor, BMJ editorial and Nick Morgan, Senior Development Editor at Blackwell Publishing who converted the authors' words and pictures into the book that is before you. Such a comprehensive review has been time consuming. I continue to be grateful for the support of my colleagues in the Edinburgh Breast Unit, and to my family Pam, Oliver, and Jonathan. I also thank the many patients who agreed to be photographed for this book, but more importantly, for the inspiration they provide in how they cope, not only with their disease but with all that we do to them.

The care provided for patients with breast cancer is better coordinated and more truly multidisciplinary than that for any other cancer. This is a testimony to those multidisciplinary teams that treat breast cancer, and to the many groups and individual women who have demanded access to good quality care for all. As a clinician I hope that the knowledge and understanding gained through research will continue to result in improved treatments. Many challenges remain in the field of breast diseases, and there is much we do not know. This book is our effort to inform you of everything that we think we know and understand about breast diseases and its management.

J Michael Dixon
Edinburgh
2005

1 Symptoms, assessment, and guidelines for referral

JM Dixon, J Thomas

One woman in four is referred to a breast clinic at some time in her life. A breast lump, which may be painful, and breast pain constitute over 80% of the breast problems that require hospital referral, and breast problems constitute up to a quarter of all women in the general surgical workload.

> When a patient presents with a breast problem the basic question for the general practitioner is, "Is there a chance that cancer is present, and, if not, can I manage these symptoms myself?"

For patients presenting with a breast lump, the general practitioner should determine whether the lump is discrete or if there is nodularity whether this is asymmetrical or is part of generalised nodularity. A discrete lump stands out from the adjoining breast tissue, has definable borders, and is measurable. Localised nodularity is more ill defined, often bilateral, and tends to fluctuate with the menstrual cycle. About 10% of all breast cancers present as asymmetrical nodularity rather than a discrete mass. When the patient is sure there is a localised lump or lumpiness, a single normal clinical examination by a general practitioner is not enough to exclude underlying disease. Reassessment after menstruation or hospital referral should be considered in all such women.

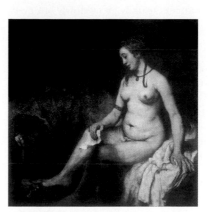

Bathsheba bathing by Rembrandt. Much discussion surrounds the shadowing on her left breast and if this represents an underlying malignancy (with permission of the Bridgeman Art Library)

Prevalence (%) of presenting symptoms in patients attending a breast clinic

- Breast lump—36%
- Painful lump or lumpiness—33%
- Pain alone—17.5%
- Nipple discharge—5%
- Nipple retraction—3%
- Strong family history of breast cancer—3%
- Breast distortion—1%
- Swelling or inflammation—1%
- Scaling nipple (eczema)—0.5%

Conditions that require hospital referral

Lump

- Any new discrete lump
- New lump in pre-existing nodularity
- Asymmetrical nodularity in a postmenopausal woman
- Asymmetric nodularity in a premenopausal woman that persists at review after menstruation
- Abscess or breast inflammation that does not settle after one course of antibiotics
- Cyst persistently refilling or recurrent cyst (if the patient has recurrent multiple cysts and the GP has the necessary skills, then aspiration is acceptable)
- Palpable or enlarged axillary mass including an enlarged axillary lymph node

Pain

- If pain is associated with a lump
- Intractable pain that interferes with a patient's lifestyle or sleep and that has failed to respond to reassurance, simple measures such as wearing a well supporting bra, and common drugs
- Unilateral persistent pain in postmenopausal women

Nipple discharge

- All women aged ≥50
- Women aged <50 with:
  Bloodstained discharge
  Spontaneous single duct discharge
  Bilateral discharge sufficient to stain clothes

Nipple retraction or distortion, nipple eczema

Change in skin contour

Family history

- Request for assessment of a woman with a strong family history of breast cancer (refer to a family cancer genetics clinic where possible)

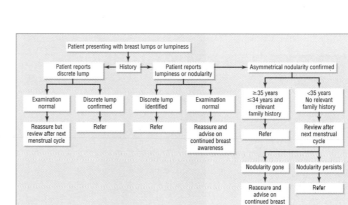

Management of patient presenting in primary care with a breast lump or localised lumpy area or nodularity

Patients who can be managed, at least initially, by their GP include

- Young women with tender, nodular breasts or older women with symmetrical nodularity, provided that they have no localised abnormality
- Young women with asymmetrical localised nodularity; these women require assessment after their next menstrual cycle, if nodularity persists hospital referral is then indicated
- Women with minor and moderate degrees of breast pain who do not have a discrete palpable lesion
- Women aged <50 who have nipple discharge that is small in amount AND is from more than one duct and is intermittent (occurs less than twice per week) and is not bloodstained. These patients should be reviewed in 2–3 weeks and if symptom persists hospital referral is indicated

Assessment of symptoms

Patient's history

Details of risk factors, including family history and current medication, should be obtained and recorded. Duration of a symptom can be helpful as cancers usually grow slowly but cysts may appear overnight.

Clinical examination

Inspection should take place in a good light with the patient's arms by her side, above her head, then pressing on her hips. Skin dimpling or a change in contour is present in up to a quarter of symptomatic patients with breast cancer. Although usually associated with an underlying malignancy, skin dimpling can follow surgery or trauma, be associated with benign conditions, or occur as part of breast involution.

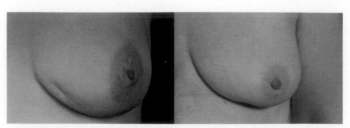

Skin dimpling (left) and change in breast contour (right) associated with underlying breast carcinoma

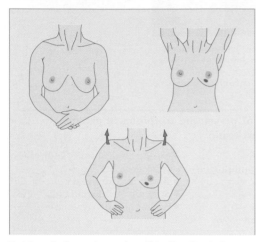

Positions for breast inspection. Skin dimpling in lower part of breast evident only when arms are elevated or pectoral muscles contracted

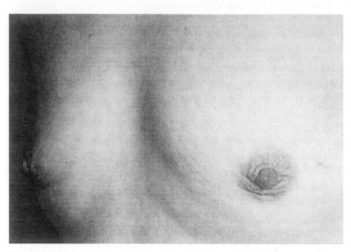

Skin dimpling visible in both breasts due to breast involution

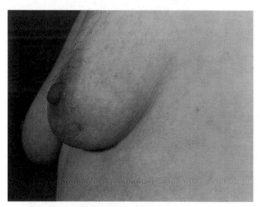

Skin dimpling after previous breast surgery

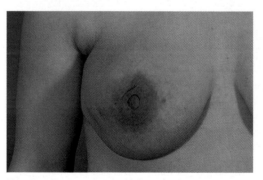

Skin dimpling associated with breast infection

Breast palpation is performed with the patient lying flat with her arms above her head, and all the breast tissue is examined using the most sensitive part of the hand, the fingertips. It is essential for the woman to have her hands under her head to spread the breast out over the chest wall because it reduces the depth of breast tissue between your hands and the chest wall and makes abnormal areas much easier to detect and define. If an abnormality is identified, it should then be assessed for contour, texture, and any deep fixation by tensing the pectoralis major, which is accomplished by asking the patient to press her hands on her hips. All palpable lesions should be measured with calipers. A clear diagram of any breast abnormalities, including dimensions and the exact position, should be recorded in the medical notes.

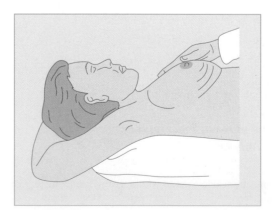

Breast palpation

Patients with breast pain should also be examined with the woman lying on each side and the underlying chest wall palpated for areas of tenderness. Much of so called breast pain emanates from the underlying chest wall.

Assessment of axillary nodes
Once both breasts have been palpated the nodal areas in the axillary and supraclavicular regions are checked. Clinical assessment of axillary nodes is often inaccurate: palpable nodes can be identified in up to 30% of patients with no clinically significant breast or other disease, and up to 40% of patients with breast cancer who have clinically normal axillary nodes actually have axillary nodal metastases.

Mammography
Mammography requires compression of the breast between two plates and is uncomfortable. Two views—oblique and craniocaudal—are usually obtained. With modern film screens a dose of less than 1.5 mGy is standard. Mammography allows detection of mass lesions, areas of parenchymal distortion, and microcalcifications. Breasts are relatively radiodense, so in younger women aged <35, mammography is of more limited value and should not be performed in younger women unless there is suspicion on clinical examination or on cytology or core biopsy that the patient has a cancer. All patients with breast cancer proved by cytology or biopsy, regardless of age, should undergo mammography before surgery for assessment of the extent of disease.

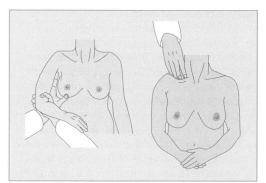
Assessment of regional nodes

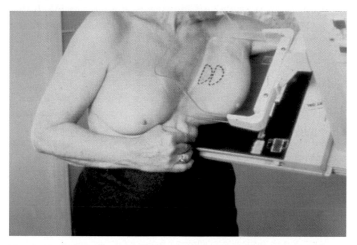
Mammography

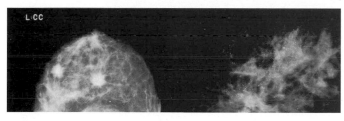
Mammograms showing (left) two mass lesions in left breast, irregular in outline with characteristics of carcinomas, and (right) mass lesion with extensive branching, impalpable microcalcification characteristic of carcinoma in situ

Ultrasonography
High frequency sound waves are beamed through the breast, and reflections are detected and turned into images. Cysts show up as transparent objects, and other benign lesions tend to have well demarcated edges whereas cancers usually have indistinct outlines. Blood flow to lesions can be imaged with colour flow Doppler ultrasound. Malignant lesions tend to have a greater blood flow than benign lesions, but the sensitivity and specificity of colour Doppler is insufficient to accurately differentiate benign from malignant lesions. Ultrasound contrast agents are available, but they are of doubtful value and not often used.

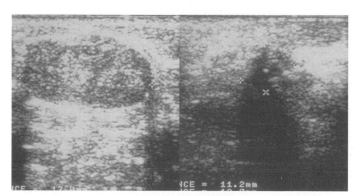
Ultrasound scans showing clear edges of fibroadenoma (left) and indistinct outline of carcinoma (right)

Magnetic resonance imaging (MRI)
Magnetic resonance imaging is an accurate way of imaging the breast. It has a high sensitivity for breast cancer and is valuable in demonstrating the extent of invasive and non-invasive disease. Ongoing studies are evaluating its role in improving the rate of successful breast conserving procedures. It is useful in the treated, conserved breast to determine whether a mammographic lesion at the site of surgery is due to scar or recurrence. It has been shown to be a valuable screening tool for high risk women between the ages of 35 and 50. MRI is the optimum method for imaging breast implants. It is also of value in assessing early response to neoadjuvant therapy in women with established breast cancer.

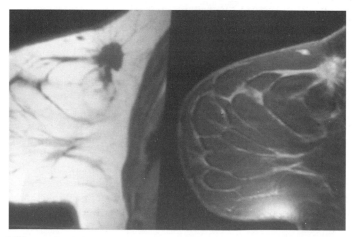
MRI scan showing cancer

Fine needle aspiration (FNA) cytology

Needle aspiration can differentiate between solid and cystic lesions. Aspiration of solid lesions requires skill to obtain enough cells for cytological analysis, and skill is needed to interpret the smears. Image guidance increases accuracy, particularly in small lesions. A 21 or 23 gauge needle attached to a syringe is introduced into the lesion and suction is applied by withdrawing the plunger; multiple passes are made through the lesion. The plunger is then released, and the material is spread onto microscope slides. These are then either air dried or sprayed with a fixative, depending on the cytologist's preference, and are stained. In some units a report is available within 30 minutes.

Touch prep cytology of core biopsy samples and sentinel lymph nodes is possible and allows immediate reporting. If the biopsy sample contains tumour this technique is very accurate. Sensitivity of touch prep cytology of lymph nodes approaches 90%, which is better than the sensitivity of frozen section.

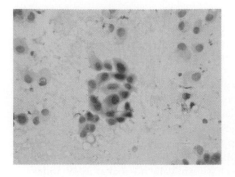

Smear from fine needle aspirate showing malignant cells that are poorly cohesive and have large polymorphic nuclei

Core biopsy

Local anaesthetic containing adrenaline solution is infiltrated into the overlying skin and surrounding breast tissue. After a minimum of 7–8 minutes, through a single small skin incision, cores of tissue are removed from the clinical mass or the area of mammographic or ultrasound abnormality by means of a cutting needle technique. A 14 gauge needle combined with a mechanical gun produces satisfactory samples and allows the procedure to be performed single handed. For calcification at least three cores need to contain the target calcification or five calcifications need to be visible in the cores to ensure adequate sampling. For mass lesions the number of cores required is less clear but with adequate local anaesthesia the procedure is painless, so multiple cores (three or more) are usually taken to ensure adequate sampling of all parts of the lesion.

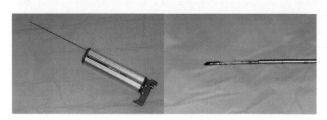

Core biopsy gun (left) and core needle with specimen (right)

Open biopsy

Open biopsy is now rarely required to establish a histopathological diagnosis except in the screening setting. All women undergoing open biopsy should have been assessed by imaging and fine needle aspiration cytology or core biopsy, or both. Women who are told that investigations have shown their lesion to be benign do not often request excision.

Breast biopsy is not without morbidity. A fifth of patients develop either a further lump under the scar or pain specifically related to the biopsy site.

> **Vacuum assisted core biopsy devices are now available, and these allow 11 or 8 gauge cores of tissue to be obtained, allowing more extensive sampling without the need to withdraw the needle from the breast. They seem to be more accurate than 14 gauge core biopsy in sampling microcalcifications**

Frozen section

Frozen section should be rarely, if ever, used to diagnose breast cancer and then should only be used to confirm a cytological diagnosis of breast cancer in a patient with clear evidence of cancer in whom core biopsy has failed to establish cancer and when a one stage surgical procedure is planned. Before proceeding to definitive surgery the patient should have been told that her lesion is considered to be malignant and have been appropriately counselled, and have had time to consider treatment options.

Its use has also been reported in assessment of excision margins after a wide local excision to ensure complete excision and assessment of axillary lymph nodes, particularly sentinel nodes, during operation to identify patients who are node positive and who may require only axillary dissection.

In both these instances reported sensitivity varies between 66 and 90%. Use of immunohistochemistry and multiple frozen sections improves sensitivity but considerably increases both

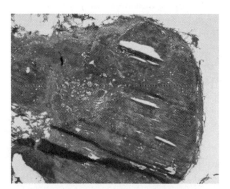

Frozen section of an axillary lymph node. It was reported as showing no evidence of metastases and this was confirmed on the subsequent paraffin section

> **The routine use of frozen section to diagnose breast cancer is no longer acceptable**

costs and the length of time to get a definitive result. Imprint cytology of sentinel nodes has a higher sensitivity and seems a better alternative to frozen section.

Accuracy of investigations

False positive results occur with all diagnostic techniques. It is acceptable to plan treatment on the basis of malignant cytology supported by a diagnosis of malignancy on clinical examination and imaging. Cytology has a false positive rate of 0.2–0.5%; the lesions most likely to be misinterpreted are fibroadenomas, papillary lesions, and areas of breast that have been irradiated. For this reason a histological diagnosis is now considered necessary to proceed with mastectomy or axillary clearance, or both. Cytology also has a false negative rate of 4–5%. Core biopsy has the advantage of providing a histological diagnosis and can differentiate between invasive and in situ carcinoma. Errors with core biopsy occur with geographical misses and inadequate sampling. Image guidance, taking images to show the needle in the lesion, and taking multiple cores is recommended to maximise sensitivity.

The sensitivity of clinical examination and mammography varies with age; only two thirds of cancers in women aged <50 are deemed suspicious or definitely malignant on clinical examination or mammography. Breast cancer in women <40 is a particular problem as it often presents with asymmetric nodularity rather than a discrete lump.

Accuracy of investigations in diagnosis of symptomatic breast disease in specialist breast clinics

	Sensitivity for cancers*	Specificity for benign disease†	PPV for cancers‡
Clinical examination	86%	90%	95%
Mammography	86%	90%	95%
Ultrasonography	90%	92%	95%
MRI	98%	75%	80%
Fine needle aspiration cytology	95%	95%	99.8%
Core biopsy	85–98%§	95%	100%

*% of invasive cancers detected by test as malignant or probably malignant (that is, complete sensitivity)

†% of benign disease detected by test as benign

‡% of lesions diagnosed as malignant that are cancers (that is, absolute PPV (positive predictive value))

§Sensitivity increase if core biopsy is image guarded

Advantages and disadvantages of techniques for assessment of breast masses

Technique	Advantages	Disadvantages
Clinical examination	Easy to perform	Low sensitivity in women ≤50
Mammography	Useful for screening women aged ≥50	Requires dedicated equipment and experienced personnel
		Low sensitivity in women ≤50
		Unpleasant (causes discomfort or actual pain)
Ultrasonography	Same sensitivity in all ages	Operator dependent
	Useful in assessing impalpable lesions	No more sensitive than mammography
	Painless	
MRI	High sensitivity in all ages	Costly—time consuming
	Accurately assesses size of cancer	Claustrophobic—low specificity
Fine needle aspiration cytology	Cheap	Operator dependent
	High sensitivity	Needs experienced cytopathologist
	Provides differential diagnosis in most instances	Painful
	Low incidence of false positives	Cannot differentiate invasive from in situ cancer
	Can be reported immediately	
Core biopsy	Easy to perform	Operator dependent
	Less painful than FNA	Cannot easily be reported immediately
	High sensitivity, particularly if image guided	Uncomfortable but less painful than FNA
	Provides a definitive histological diagnosis	Bruising and swelling
	Almost zero false positive rate	

Triple assessment

This is the combination of clinical examination, imaging (usually mammography with or without ultrasonography for women aged ≥35 and ultrasonography alone for women aged <35), and fine needle aspiration cytology or core biopsy, or both.

Delay in diagnosis

Delay in the diagnosis of breast cancer is a common reason for patients taking legal action against medical practitioners. Currently 1.5–4 % of patients with breast cancer experience a diagnostic delay of eight weeks or longer. Diagnostic delay is a particular problem in younger women, because cancers in these younger women often manifest as localised nodularity rather

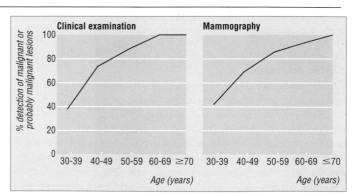

Sensitivity of clinical examination and mammography by age in patients presenting with a breast mass. Adapted from Dixon JM et al. *Br J Surg* 1984; 71:593–6

than a discrete lump. For this reason all women who have either discrete lumps or localised areas of asymmetric nodularity should have triple assessment. The doctor who ordered the investigations should check all the reports, which should be filed in the patient's notes. Details of clinical findings must be recorded legibly in the patient's records and include a diagram marking all areas of abnormality and a doctor's signature.

One stop clinics

In a patient with a discrete breast mass or a localised area of nodularity some centres offer immediate reporting of imaging and cytology from a fine needle aspirate or touch preparation from a core biopsy sample. One stop clinics have advantages for women with benign lumps, who can be reassured and discharged after a single visit; they are only cost effective in centres that see many patients.

Investigation of breast symptoms

Breast mass and localised nodularity

All patients should be assessed by triple assessment. It is not necessary to excise all solid breast masses, and a selective policy is recommended on the basis of the results of triple assessment. Core biopsy, preferably image guided, has replaced cytology as the most commonly used diagnostic investigation. Combining FNA and core biopsy increases sensitivity obtained with each investigation alone. Combining FNA and core biopsy or using core biopsy alone with touch preparation or roll cytology allows both immediate reporting and a histological diagnosis.

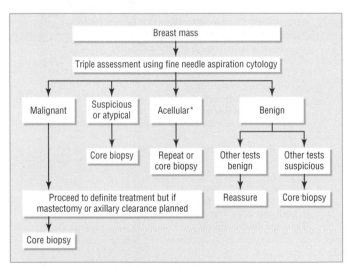

Investigation of a breast mass using fine needle aspiration as initial investigation (*acellular aspirates are not always inadequate specimens and in the presence of lucent breasts may be enough to exclude malignancy)

Nipple discharge

Treatment depends on whether the discharge is spontaneous and whether it is from one or several ducts. Single duct discharge should be checked by testing for haemoglobin. Only moderate or large amounts of blood are significant. About 5–10% of patients with bloodstained discharge will be found to have an underlying malignancy. Most bloodstained discharges are due to simple papillomas or other benign conditions. All patients with spontaneous discharge should have clinical examination and, if aged >35, mammography. Ductography and ductoscopy can localise lesions and may have a role in

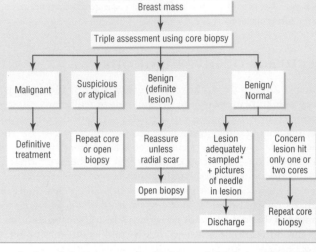

Investigation of a breast mass or localised area of nodularity with core biopsy (*minimum of three cores are required, preferably image guided, to be certain that lesion is adequately sampled)

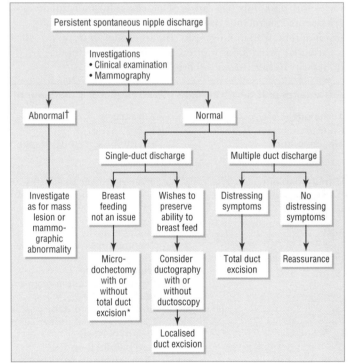

Investigation of nipple discharge (*some surgeons prefer total duct excision in women aged >45 to reduce incidence of discharge from other ducts)

†If lesion on mammograms is incidental and unlikely to be related to nipple discharge combine with investigation of single or multiple duct discharge as appropriate

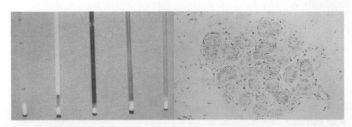

Physiological breast secretions collected from non-pregnant women (left). Note range of colours from white to blue-black. Physiological secretions visible in a normal breast lobule (right)

young women to direct and limit any excision in an effort to maintain the ability to breast feed. Physiological nipple discharge is common: two thirds of premenopausal women can be made to produce nipple secretion by cleansing the nipple and applying suction. This physiological discharge varies in colour from white to yellow to green to blue-black.

Galactorrhoea is copious bilateral milky discharge not associated with pregnancy or breastfeeding. Prolactin levels are usually but not always raised in women with galactorrhoea. A careful drug history should be taken as various drugs, particularly psychotropic agents, can cause hyperprolactinaemia. In the absence of relevant drugs, a search for a pituitary tumour should be instituted in a patient with a raised prolactin >1000 IU/l.

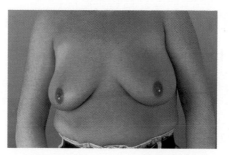
Galactorrhoea

Blocked Montgomery's tubercle

Montgomery's tubercles are blind-ending ducts in the areola. Secretions from the lining cells may become inspissated and present as a periareolar lump that can be locally excised if troublesome. They can become infected.

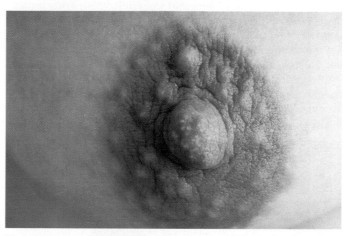
Blocked Montgomery's tubercle

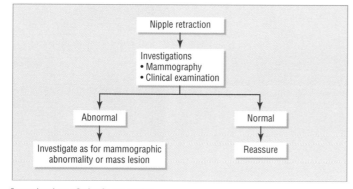
Investigation of nipple retraction

Nipple retraction

Slit-like retraction of the nipple is characteristic of benign disease, whereas nipple inversion, when the whole nipple is pulled in, occurs in association with both breast cancer and inflammatory breast conditions. For patients with congenital nipple retraction and acquired nipple retraction, which is unsightly and does not respond to conservative measures, such as suction devices or nipple shields, surgery including duct division or excision can be successful at everting the nipple. Women need to be informed duct excision can result in loss of ability to breast feed and loss or reduction of nipple sensation or sometimes nipple hypersensitivity.

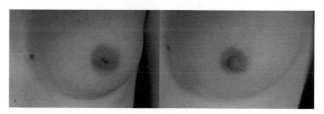
Before and after surgery for nipple eversion

Breast pain

Cyclical breast pain should be differentiated from non-cyclical pain, and its severity should be assessed by means of a careful history and clinical examination. Mammography or ultrasonography, or both, is indicated in patients with unilateral persistent mastalgia or a localised area of painful nodularity. Focal lesions should be investigated with fine needle aspiration cytology or core biopsy, or both.

Indications for excision of a breast lesion

- Diagnosis of malignancy on cytology not confirmed by subsequent core biopsy when a mastectomy or axillary clearance is planned
- Diagnosis of atypical hyperplasia on core biopsy
- Radial scar: diagnosed by imaging and core biopsy
- Indeterminate papillary lesions
- Suspicion of malignancy on one or more investigations with indeterminate or inadequate core biopsy
- Request by patient for excision

Further reading

- Dixon JM. Indications and techniques of breast biopsy. *Curr Prac Surg* 1993;5:142–8.
- Berg WA, Guttierrez L, Ness Avier MS, Carter WB, Bhargavan M, Lewis RS, et al. Diagnostic accuracy of mammography, clinical examination, US and MR imaging in preoperative assessment of breast cancer. *Radiology* 2004:233:830–49.
- Hughes LE, Mansel RE, Webster DJT. *Benign disorders and diseases of the breast: concepts and clinical management*. 2nd ed. London: Saunders, 2000.

- Helvie MA. Mammography in diseases of the breast. In: Harris JR, Lippman ME, Morrow M, Osborne CK, eds. *Imaging analysis*. Philadelphia: Lippincott Williams and Wilkins, 2004:131–48.
- Mendelson EB. Ultrasonographic imaging in diseases of the breast. In: Harris JR, Lippman ME, Morrow M, Osborne CK, eds. *Imaging analysis*. Philadelphia: Lippincott Williams and Wilkins, 2004:149–63.
- Orel SG. Magnetic resonance imaging in diseases of the breast. In: Harris JR, Lippman ME, Morrow M, Osborne CK, eds. *Imaging analysis*. Philadelphia: Lippincott Williams and Wilkins, 2004:165–79.

2 Congenital problems and aberrations of normal development and involution

JM Dixon, J Thomas

Congenital abnormalities

Extra nipples and breasts

Between 1% and 5% of men and women have supernumerary or accessory nipples or, less commonly, supernumerary or accessory breasts. These usually develop along the milk line: the most common site for accessory nipples is just below the normal breast, and the most common site for accessory breast tissue is the lower axilla. Accessory breasts below the umbilicus are extremely rare. Extra breasts or nipples rarely require treatment unless they are unsightly, although they are subject to the same diseases as normal breasts and nipples.

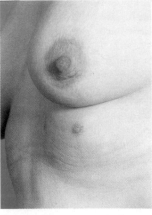

Patient with accessory nipple

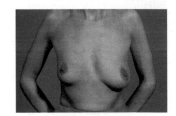

Usual sites of accessory nipples and breast along milk lines

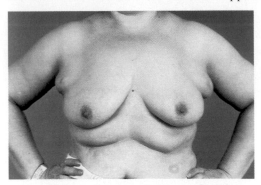

Patient with bilateral accessory breasts

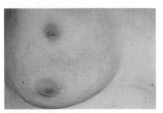

Patient with two nipples in one breast: One normal, and the other accessory

Absence or hypoplasia of the breast

One breast can be absent or hypoplastic, usually in association with defects in one or both pectoral muscles. Some degree of breast asymmetry is usual, and the left breast is more commonly larger than the right. True breast asymmetry can be treated by augmentation of the smaller breast, reduction or elevation of the larger breast, or a combination of procedures.

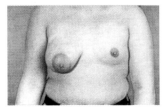

Left breast hypoplasia

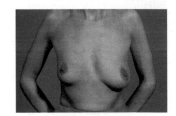

Breast asymmetry

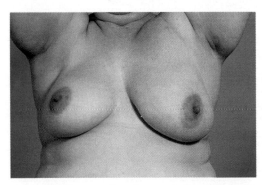
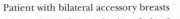

Absence of left pectoralis major muscle but normal right breast

Chest wall abnormalities

About 90% of patients with true unilateral absence of a breast have either absence or hypoplasia of the pectoral muscles. In contrast, 90% of patients with pectoral muscle defects have normal breasts. Some patients have abnormalities of the pectoral muscles and absence or hypoplasia of the breast associated with a characteristic deformity of the upper limb. This cluster of anomalies is called Poland's syndrome. Abnormalities of the chest wall, such as pectus excavatum, and deformities of the thoracic spine, such as scoliosis, can also result in normal symmetrical breasts seeming asymmetrical.

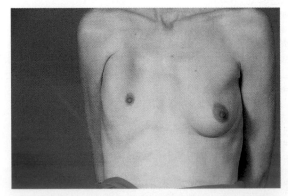

Poland's syndrome with hypoplasia of right breast and absent chest wall muscles (patient also had typical hand abnormality)

Breast development and involution

The breast is identical in boys and girls until puberty. Growth begins at about the age of 10 and may initially be asymmetrical: a unilateral breast lump in a 9–10 year old girl is invariably a developing breast, and biopsy specimens should not be taken from girls of this age as this can damage the breast bud. The functional unit of the breast is the terminal duct lobular unit or lobule, which drains via a branching duct system to the nipple. The duct system does not run in a truly radial manner, and the breast is not separated into easily defined segments. The lobules and ducts—the glandular tissue—are supported by fibrous tissue—the stroma. Most benign breast conditions and almost all breast cancers arise within the terminal duct lobular unit.

After the breast has developed, it undergoes regular changes related to the menstrual cycle. Pregnancy results in a doubling of the breast weight at term, and the breast involutes after pregnancy. In nulliparous women breast involution begins at some time after the age of 30. During involution the breast stroma is replaced by fat so that the breast becomes less radiodense, softer, and ptotic (droopy). Changes in the glandular tissue include the development of areas of fibrosis, the formation of small cysts (microcysts), and an increase in the number of glandular elements (adenosis). The life cycle of the breast consists of three main periods: development (and early reproductive life), mature reproductive life, and involution. Most benign breast conditions occur during one specific period and are so common that they are best considered as aberrations rather than disease.

Aberrations of breast development

Juvenile or virginal hypertrophy
Prepubertal breast enlargement is common and requires investigation only if it is associated with other signs of sexual maturation. Uncontrolled overgrowth of breast tissue can occur in adolescent girls whose breasts develop normally during puberty but then continue to grow, often quite rapidly. No endocrine abnormality can be detected in these girls.

Patients present with social embarrassment, pain, discomfort, and inability to perform regular daily tasks. Reduction mammoplasty considerably improves their quality of life and should be more widely available.

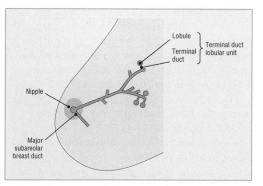

Anatomy of breast showing terminal duct lobular units and branching system of ducts

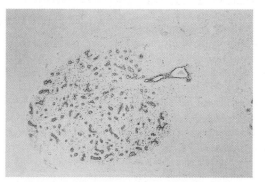

Terminal duct lobular unit

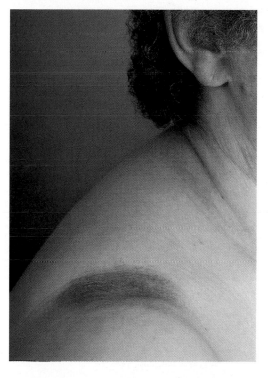

Shoulder indentation resulting from bra strap in juvenile hypertrophy

Aberrations of normal breast development and involution

Age (years)	Normal process	Aberration
<25	Breast development: • Stromal • Lobular	Juvenile hypertrophy Fibroadenoma
25–40	Cyclical activity	Cyclical mastalgia; cyclical nodularity (diffuse or focal)
35–55	Involution: • Lobular • Stromal • Ductal	Macrocysts Sclerosing lesions Duct ectasia

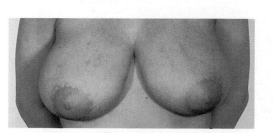

Patient with juvenile hypertrophy before surgery

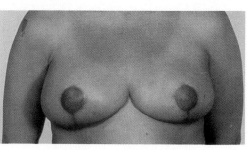

Patient with juvenile hypertrophy after surgery

Fibroadenoma

Although classified in most textbooks as benign neoplasms, fibroadenomas are best considered as aberrations of normal development: they develop from a whole lobule and not from a single cell, they are common, and they are under the same hormonal control as the rest of the breast tissue. Fibroadenomas account for about 13% of all palpable symptomatic breast masses, but in women aged ≤20 they account for almost 60% of such masses. There are three separate types of fibroadenoma: common fibroadenoma, giant fibroadenoma, and juvenile fibroadenoma. There is no universally accepted definition of what constitutes a giant fibroadenoma, but most consider that it should measure over 5 cm in diameter. Juvenile fibroadenomas occur in adolescent girls and sometimes undergo rapid growth but are managed in the same way as the common fibroadenoma.

Phyllodes tumours are distinct pathological entities. They are usually larger than fibroadenomas, occur in an older age group, have malignant potential, and cannot always be differentiated clinically from fibroadenomas. Phyllodes tumours focally have an infiltrative margin and form a spectrum from benign (80%) to malignant (20%). About 20% of benign phyllodes tumours recur after excision.

Fibroadenomas have characteristic mammographic features in older patients when they calcify. A few patients have multiple fibroadenomas. Over a two year period less than 10% of common fibroadenomas increase in size, about one third get smaller or completely disappear, and the remainder stay the same size. Fibroadenomas usually increase in size during pregnancy, sometimes dramatically. The appearance on ultrasonography also changes with fluid (milk) filled spaces, which should not be confused with the spaces seen sometimes in phyllodes tumours.

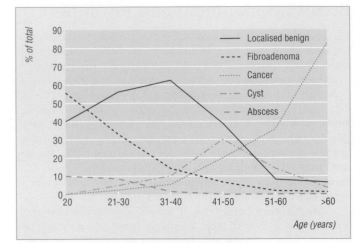
Changing frequencies of different discrete breast lumps with age

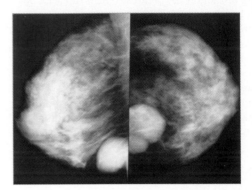
Mammogram of a benign phyllodes tumour

Final diagnosis in patients with palpable breast mass

Diagnosis (%)		Diagnosis (%)	
Localised benign*	38	Periductal mastitis	1
Cysts	15	Duct ectasia	1
Carcinoma	26	Abscess	1
Fibroadenoma	13	Others	5

*Localised areas of nodularity that histologically show no clinically significant abnormality or aberrations of normal involution

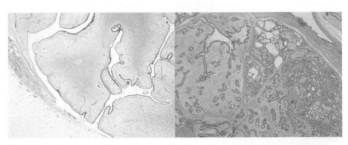
Histology of common fibroadenoma (left) and benign phyllodes tumour (right)

Management

A diagnosis based on cytology is acceptable providing the patient is young (<30) and the lesion is small (<3 cm) and has characteristic clinical and imaging features. Otherwise a histological diagnosis should be established by core biopsy. In patients with multiple fibroadenomas, two or more lesions should be sampled and the rest should be imaged and monitored.

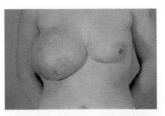
Juvenile fibroadenoma of right breast

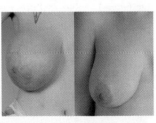
Juvenile (giant) fibroadenoma before and after surgery

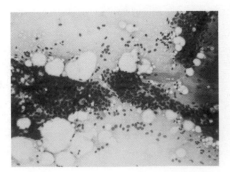
Fine needle aspirate of a fibroadenoma showing benign cells in a background of bare nuclei

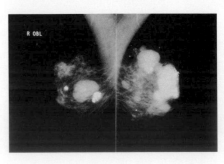
Mammograms of multiple calcified fibroadenoma

Fibroadenomas over 4 cm require full assessment by core biopsy. Multiple passes are required to ensure that the lesion is not a phyllodes tumour. Cytology alone is not recommended in these larger lesions as it is not possible on cytology to distinguish with confidence fibroadenomas from phyllodes tumours. These larger lesions should be excised with a 1 cm margin if a phyllodes tumour is suspected on core biopsy. Large juvenile fibroadenomas can be excised through inferior or inferolateral incisions, which give good cosmetic results. Common fibroadenomas diagnosed in women aged <30 by clinical examination, ultrasonography, and fine needle aspiration cytology and in older women by core biopsy require excision only if it is requested by the patient. Excision of small fibroadenomas is possible with the new vacuum assisted larger core biopsy devices, such as the 8 gauge mammotome.

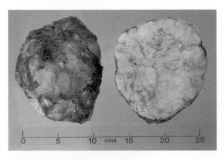

Cross section of giant fibroadenoma

Aberrations in the early reproductive period

Pain and nodularity

Cyclical pain and nodularity are so common that they can be regarded as physiological and not pathological. Severe or prolonged pain is regarded as an aberration. Focal breast nodularity is the most common cause of a breast lump and is seen in women of all ages. When excised, most of these areas of nodularity show either no pathological abnormality or aberrations of the normal involutional process such as focal areas of fibrosis or sclerosis. The preferred pathological term is benign breast change, and terms such as fibroadenosis, fibrocystic disease, and mastitis should no longer be used by clinicians or pathologists.

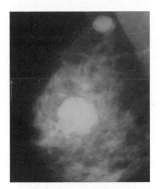

Mammogram of patient with cyst and cancer

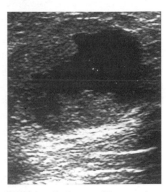

Ultrasound picture of intracystic cancer

Aberrations of involution

Palpable breast cysts

About 7% of women in Western countries will present at some time in their life with a palpable breast cyst. Palpable cysts constitute 15% of all discrete breast masses. Cysts are distended and involuted lobules and are most common in perimenopausal women. Most present as a smooth discrete breast lump that can be painful and is sometimes visible.

Cysts have characteristic halos on mammography and are readily diagnosed by ultrasonography. The diagnosis can also be established by needle aspiration, and providing the fluid is not bloodstained it should not be sent for cytology. After aspiration the breast should be re-examined to check that the palpable mass has disappeared. Any residual mass requires full assessment, including mammography. About 1–3% of patients presenting with cysts have carcinomas; most of these are not associated with the cyst but are incidental findings on ultrasonography or mammography.

Patients with cysts have a slightly increased risk of developing breast cancer (twice to three times the risk), but the magnitude of this risk is not clinically significant.

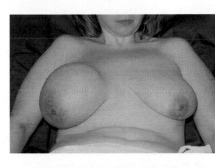

Patient with intracystic cancer of the right breast

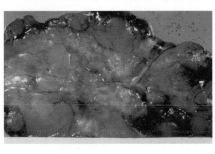

Excision specimen sliced to show area of sclerosis (histologically confirmed)

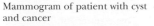

The mammographic appearance of sclerosing lesions mimics that of cancer, causing diagnostic problems during breast screening

Sclerosis

Aberrations of stromal involution include the development of localised areas of excessive fibrosis or sclerosis. Pathologically, these lesions can be separated into three groups: sclerosing adenosis, radial scars, and complex sclerosing lesions (this term incorporates lesions previously called sclerosing papillomatosis and includes infiltrating epitheliosis).

They are clinically important because of the diagnostic problems they cause during breast screening. Excision biopsy is often required to make a definitive diagnosis.

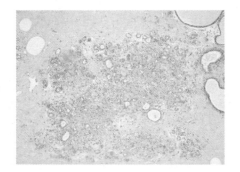

Histology of sclerosing adenosis, note the crowding of the acinar units

Duct ectasia

The major subareolar ducts dilate and shorten during involution, and, by the age of 70, 40% of women have substantial duct dilatation or duct ectasia. Some women with excessive dilatation and shortening present with nipple discharge, nipple retraction, or a palpable mass that may be hard or doughy. The discharge is usually cheesy, and the nipple retraction is classically slit-like. Surgery is indicated only if the discharge is troublesome or the patient wants the nipple to be everted.

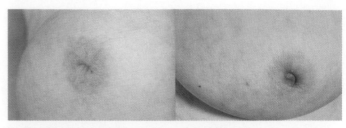

Slit-like nipple retraction due to duct ectasia (left) and nipple retraction due to breast cancer (right)

Gynaecomastia

Gynaecomastia (the growth of breast tissue in males to any extent in all ages) is entirely benign and usually reversible. It commonly occurs in puberty and old age. It is seen in 30–60% of boys aged 10–16 years and usually requires no treatment as 80% resolve spontaneously within two years. Embarrassment or persistent enlargement are indications for surgical referral.

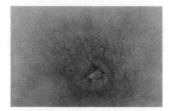

Patient with dried secretion in an inverted nipple characteristic of duct ectasia

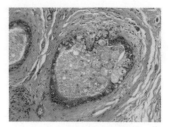

Duct ectasia showing dilated ducts but little active periductal inflammation

Causes of gynaecomastia

Cause	(%)	Cause	(%)
Puberty	25	Testicular tumours	3
Idiopathic (senescent)	25	Secondary hypogonadism	2
Drugs (including cimetidine, digoxin, spironolactone, androgens, or antioestrogens)	10–20	Hyperthyroidism	1.5
Cirrhosis or malnutrition	8	Renal disease	1
Primary hypogonadism	8		

Senescent gynaecomastia commonly affects men aged between 50 and 80, and in most it does not seem to be associated with any endocrine abnormality. A careful history and examination will often reveal the cause. A history of recent progressive breast enlargement without pain or tenderness and without an easily identifiable cause is an indication for investigation. Mammography can differentiate between breast enlargement due to fat or gynaecomastia and is valuable if malignancy is suspected. Fine needle aspiration cytology and/or core biopsy should be performed if there is clinical or mammographic suspicion of breast cancer. Only if no clear cause is apparent should blood hormone concentrations be measured.

In drug related gynaecomastia withdrawal of the drug or change to an alternative treatment should be considered. Gynaecomastia is seen in body builders who take anabolic steroids; some have learnt that by taking tamoxifen they can combat this. Both tamoxifen and danazol improve symptoms in patients with gynaecomastia but recurrence after stopping drugs can be a problem. Surgery for gynaecomastia is not easy, should follow recognised protocols, and should be performed by experienced breast or plastic surgeons.

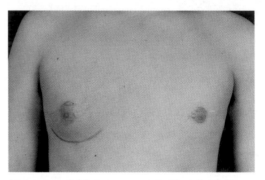

Adolescent left sided gynaecomastia. Black line indicates lower limit of dissection

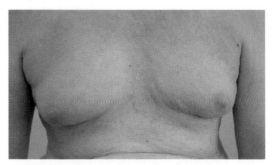

Bilateral senescent gynaecomastia

Benign neoplasms and proliferations

Epithelial hyperplasia

Epithelial hyperplasia is an increase in the number of cells lining the terminal duct lobular unit. This was previously called epitheliosis or papillomatosis, but these terms are now obsolete. The degree of hyperplasia can be graded as mild, moderate, or florid (severe).

If the hyperplastic cells also show cellular atypia the condition is called atypical hyperplasia. The absolute risk of breast cancer in a woman with atypical hyperplasia who does

> **Atypical hyperplasia is the only benign breast condition associated with a significantly increased risk of subsequent breast cancer**

not have a first degree relative with breast cancer is 8% at 10 years; for a woman with a first degree relative with breast cancer, the risk is 20–25% at 15 years.

Duct papillomas

These can be single or multiple. They are common and should probably be considered as aberrations rather than true benign neoplasms as they show minimal malignant potential. The most common symptom is nipple discharge, which is often bloodstained.

Lipomas

These soft lobulated radiolucent lesions are common in the breast. Interest in these lesions lies in the confusion with pseudolipoma, a soft mass that can be felt around a breast cancer and that is caused by indrawing of the surrounding fat by a spiculated carcinoma.

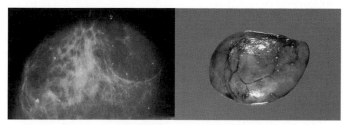

Mammogram (left) showing a large radiolucent lipoma present anteriorly and medially in breast (white mark represents lateral aspect of mammogram) and (right) the excised tumour

Nipple adenoma

This is an ulcerating lesion on the nipple that presents as a lump in the nipple or as nipple discharge. Treatment is wide excision. It is usually possible to save the nipple.

Haematomas

These most commonly follow trauma such as a road traffic incident or after fine needle aspiration, core biopsy, or open biopsy. In extremely unusual circumstances a breast carcinoma may present with a spontaneous haematoma. Breast haematoma can also occur spontaneously in patients on anticoagulant therapy.

Fat necrosis

Fat necrosis of the breast is often called "traumatic fat necrosis," though a history of trauma is present in only about 40% of patients. It is most commonly seen after road traffic incidents as a result of seat belt trauma to the breast.

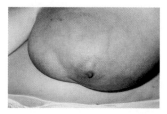

Fat necrosis of the breast after trauma caused by seat belt

Sarcoidosis

Patients with sarcoid can present with single or multiple masses within the breast. A breast mass can occur either as the first

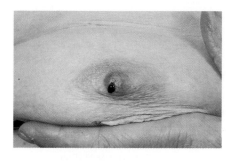

Bloodstained nipple discharge

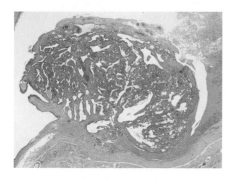

Histology of a duct papilloma that measures 5 mm

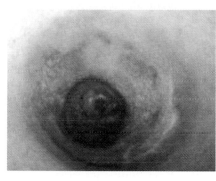

Adenoma of the nipple. There is a small nodule and a visible area of ulceration on the surface of the nipple. This patient had undergone a recent microdochectomy but the nipple adenoma had been missed and nipple discharge persisted

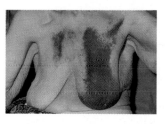

Breast haematoma

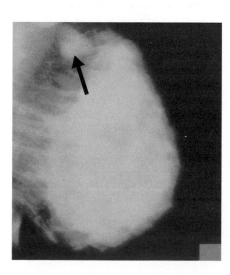

Sarcoidosis of the breast

13

presentation or can occur in a patient with sarcoidosis elsewhere. Diagnosis is confirmed by core biopsy or excision.

Other benign conditions

Mondor's disease
Thrombosis of superficial veins in the skin of the breast is known as Mondor's disease. The thoracoepigastric vein is most commonly affected. Most often seen after surgery or trauma, it can occur spontaneously particularly in patients with an underlying clotting abnormality such as factor V Leiden. It is usually painful and tender to touch. No specific treatment is required, but it can take some time to settle completely.

Hamartoma
Uncommon, they are also known as fibroadenolipomas. They consist of fibroglandular tissue admixed with fat surrounded by a capsule and present clinically as a discrete breast mass. The surrounding halo of connective tissue differentiates these lesions on imaging from fibroadenomas.

Para areola cysts
These cysts are rare and occur in pubertal and postpubertal teenagers (13–16 years) presenting as discrete superficial cystic masses at the areola margin; occasionally they become infected. They can be interpreted as solid on ultrasonography because of numerous internal echoes. Diagnosis and treatment is by aspiration, though if they cause no symptoms and ultrasonography shows a cystic lesion no intervention is required as they disappear with time.

Arteritis and aneurysm
Patients with generalised vascular disease can develop localised vasculitis involving vessels in the breast to produce a localised mass. Aneurysmal dilatation of arteries in the breast has been described and presents clinically as a discrete mass with an audible bruit on auscultation.

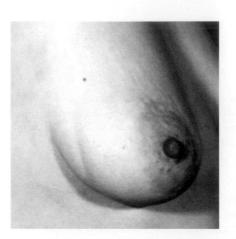

Mondor's disease of the right breast. Note the linear indentation in the breast at the site of the thrombosed vessel

Further reading

- Bostwick J. *Plastic reconstructive surgery.* St Louis, Missouri, 1990:293–408.
- Dixon JM, Dobie V, Lamb J, Walsh JS, Chetty U. Assessment of the acceptability of conservative management of fibroadenoma of the breast. *Br J Surg* 1996;83:264–5.
- Hughes LE, Mansel RE, Webster DJT. *Benign disorders and diseases of the breast: concepts and clinical management.* 2nd ed. London: Saunders, 2000.
- Osborne MP. Breast development and anatomy. In: Harris JR, Lippman ME, Morrow M, Hellman S, eds. *Diseases of the breast.* Philadelphia: Lippincott-Raven, 2004.
- Parker LN, Gray DR, Lai MK, Levin ER. Treatment of gynaecomastia with tamoxifen: a double-blind crossover study. *Metabolism* 1986;35:705–8.
- Schnitt SJ, Connolly JL. Pathology of benign breast disorders in diseases of the breast. In: Harris JR, Lippman ME, Morrow M, Osborne CK, eds. *Diseases of the breast.* Philadelphia: Lippincott Williams and Wilkins, 2004:77–99.
- Anderson BO, Lawton TJ, Lehman CD, Moe RE. Phyllodes tumor. In: Harris JR, Lippman ME, Morrow M, Osborne CK, eds. *Diseases of the breast.* Philadelphia: Lippincott Williams and Wilkins, 2004:991–1006.
- Braunstein GD. Management of gynecomastia. In: Harris JR, Lippman ME, Morrow M, Osborne CK, eds. *Diseases of the breast.* Philadelphia: Lippincott Williams and Wilkins, 2004:69–76.

3 Mastalgia

J Iddon

Mastalgia is pain in the breast. Up to 70% of women will experience this at some time during their life. The pain women describe as breast pain can arise either in the breast tissue itself or it can be referred pain, which is felt in the breast. The nerve supply to the breast is from the anterolateral and anteromedial branches of the intercostal nerves from T3 to T5 and irritation of these nerves anywhere along their course can lead to pain that is felt in the breast or nipple. Occasionally pain can be referred from the breast or chest wall through the intercostobrachial nerve to the inner aspect of the arm.

It is important to differentiate between pain referred to the breast from the chest wall and true breast pain because management of these two conditions is different. It is less important to differentiate cyclical mastalgia, in which the pain occurs only in the premenstrual part of the menstrual cycle, from non-cyclical mastalgia, in which pain may last throughout the cycle or bear no relation to the menstrual cycle, as management of these conditions is similar.

Primary care studies indicate that the most common type of mastalgia is pain referred from the chest wall, whereas in breast clinics true breast pain is said to be more common. Clinical examination reveals that even in women with a classic history of cyclical breast pain, the chest wall is often the site of origin of the pain.

Chest wall pain

Features suggesting that breast pain is referred rather than originating in the breast include pain that is unilateral, brought on by activity, is very lateral or medial in the breast, and can be reproduced by pressure on a specific area of the back or chest wall. Women who are postmenopausal and not taking hormonal supplements or who arc known to have spondylosis or osteoarthritis are more likely to have musculoskeletal pain rather than true breast pain.

Careful clinical examination is essential to help determine the site of origin of the pain. Any patient complaining of breast pain should be examined with her lying on each side, allowing the breast to fall away from the chest wall, and the underlying muscles and ribs palpated. The patient should be asked to indicate if there is any localised tenderness on palpation of the chest wall and whether any discomfort evident during examination is similar to the pain they normally experience. If the patient has pain in the lower part the breast the underlying chest wall is examined by lifting the breast with one hand while palpating the underlying chest wall with the other hand. Allowing the woman herself to confirm that the site of maximal tenderness is in the underlying chest wall rather than the breast is effective in reassuring patients that there is no significant breast problem.

Treatment of chest wall pain

The mainstay of treating chest wall pain is reassurance that there is no serious underlying cause for the pain. In women with troublesome pain, providing there are no contraindications, non-steroidal anti-inflammatory drugs (NSAIDs) are usually effective. Although there is no evidence to suggest that topical NSAIDs have any benefit over oral preparations there is some evidence that topical agents cause fewer gastrointestinal problems. Women often report a recent increase in activities, such as gardening decorating, lifting, or

---

Principles of mastalgia treatment

Exclude cancer	Assess site of pain
Clinical examination	True breast pain
Mammography in women aged >35	Chest wall pain
Ultrasonography if localised area of pain	
Provide reassurance and information	

Breast pain is a rare symptom of breast cancer. In a 10 year survey in Edinburgh of 8504 patients presenting with breast pain as their major symptom, 220 (2.7%) were subsequently diagnosed with breast cancer. During this period 4740 patients had breast cancer, which means that 4.6% of women with breast cancer had pain as an important presenting symptom

---

Classification of non-cyclical mastalgia

Chest wall causes	Non-breast causes
Such as tender costochondral junctions (Tietze's syndrome)	Cervical and thoracic spondylosis
True breast pain	Lung disease
Diffuse breast pain	Gall stones
Trigger spots in breast	Exogenous oestrogens, such as hormone replacement therapy
	Thoracic outlet syndrome

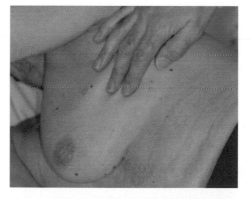

How to examine for lateral chest wall tenderness. The patient is rolled on her side with the breast falling away from the site of the pain laterally. The underlying chest wall is then palpated to identify any area of localised tenderness

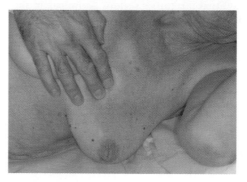

How to examine for medial chest wall tenderness over the costochondral junctions. The patient is rolled on her side with the breast falling away from the site of the pain medially. The underlying chest wall is then palpated to identify any area of localised tenderness

increased visits to the gym, after which they become aware of the pain. Infiltrating the affected chest wall with prednisolone 40 mg in depot form combined with long acting local anaesthetic can effectively treat patients with an area of tenderness localised to a specific area in the chest wall. If the correct area has been targeted pain relief should follow quickly. About half of women get long lasting benefit from a single injection. Repeating the injection after 4–6 weeks increases both the number of women getting benefit and provides long lasting pain control for two thirds of women with troublesome pain that "interferes" with regular daily activities.

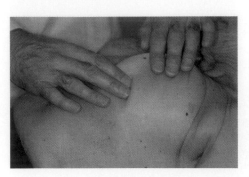

How to examine for chest wall tenderness under the lower part of the breast. The breast is lifted upwards by one hand while the other hand presses gently on the underlying chest wall to identify any area of localised tenderness

True mastalgia

Pain arising in the breast tissue itself is often associated with cyclical swelling and nodularity. Hormonal changes are thought to be responsible for these changes in the breast as they are most commonly seen in the week before menstruation and are relieved by its onset. In addition the pain can be brought on by hormonal manipulation such as oestrogen containing hormone replacement therapy. It is much less of a problem with tibolone. There are several theories regarding the pathophysiology of mastalgia.

Too much oestrogen—Measurements of serum oestrogen concentrations have not shown any differences between women with pain and normal controls.

Not enough progesterone—A single study has shown reduced serum progesterone concentration in the luteal phase in women with mastalgia when compared with controls.

Too much prolactin—Measuring prolactin is complicated because of diurnal variation in hormone levels. Measurement of 24 hour serum prolactin profiles and of tissue concentrations of prolactin in breast biopsy samples taken either during the day or night have not shown any differences between women with and without mastalgia. The prolactin response after stimulation has been studied, and women with mastalgia produced more prolactin for longer, suggesting that there may be a problem in the prolactin pathway at the level of the hypothalamus.

Increased receptor sensitivity in breast tissue/abnormal fatty acids—Women with mastalgia have different fatty acid profiles to women without pain in that they have an increased ratio of saturated fatty acids to essential fatty acids. Cell membranes that have a high proportion of saturated fats become rigid and membrane receptors are easier for ligands to bind to. If cell membranes are composed of unsaturated fats, they are more fluid, and receptors can be enveloped in folds of the membrane making it harder for ligands to access and stimulate the receptor. Because women with mastalgia have more saturated fatty acids the oestrogen receptor is more available making the cells in the breast more sensitive to the effects of oestrogen.

Treatments for mastalgia

Reassurance

Breast pain often causes women to seek medical attention because they are afraid that it signifies serious pathology in the breast. Non-randomised studies have shown that reassurance is effective management in 70% of women.

Non-specific measures

Pain in bed at night is a problem for many women with both chest wall pain and true mastalgia. Wearing a soft supportive bra at night stops the breast pulling down on the chest wall, supports tender breast tissue, and helps many women to sleep.

There are reports that avoiding caffeine in drinks such as tea, coffee, and cola improves breast pain, but these are anecdotal and there is no convincing evidence that caffeine is

Outcome in women with chest wall pain treated by local infiltration of bupivacaine (Marcain) plus depot steroid (injected group) or observation alone (comparative group)

	Injected group	Comparative group
No of women	104	34
No who attended follow up	100	29
No (%) with complete resolution of pain*	61* (61)	5 (17)
No (%) with partial resolution of pain	22 (22)	8 (22.5)
No (%) with successful outcome*	83* (83)	13 (44.8)

*Differences significant at P < 0.0001

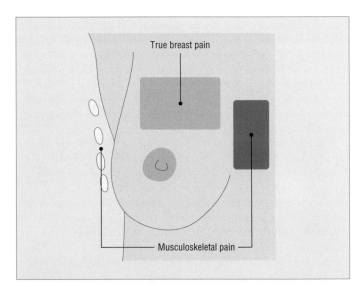

Classification of non-cyclical breast pain. Non-cyclical pain can be divided into true breast pain arising from the breast tissue or musculoskeletal pain arising from the ribs or chest wall. Musculoskeletal pain is commonly medially (Tietze's syndrome) or laterally at the edge of the breast

Researchers have suggested that some women get breast pain because of overstimulation of breast cells by methylxanthines as a result of high caffeine intake. However, one study found identical serum caffeine concentrations in women with and without mastalgia, and randomised trials have also failed to demonstrate a benefit for caffeine restriction. Any association between mastalgia and caffeine intake thus remains unproved

important in the aetiology of breast pain. For chest wall pain, gentle exercise and stretching of the muscles, such as provided by swimming, seems sensible and is advised by some, but this has not been studied.

Evening primrose oil (EPO), γ linoleic acid (GLA), efamast
Preparations containing GLA were used in the treatment of mastalgia until October 2002, when they were withdrawn from prescription by the medicines control agency as they viewed there was no good evidence to support their use. Two double blind randomised controlled trials of EPO compared with placebo have been conducted and published. Neither study showed any difference between treatment and control groups. There was a reported improvement in symptoms early during the first three months of treatment and a worsening of symptoms after crossover, regardless of whether patients received treatment or placebo first. A further study published in abstract form showed improvement in pain scores in the treated group for both cyclical and non-cyclical pain, but this study did not report results after crossover and there was a high drop out rate in the placebo arm. Other studies have been published but these were not randomised or blinded.

Low fat diet
Two randomised controlled studies have shown that a low fat diet is effective in improving cyclical mastalgia. Both studies limited the dietary fat intake to less than 15% of calories, and patients who responded showed changes in their serum lipid profiles. These studies were not blinded so a placebo effect cannot be excluded. Such low fat diets are difficult to maintain for longer than a few weeks.

Danazol
One double blind randomised controlled trial of danazol 200 mg/day compared with placebo showed a significant improvement in breast pain. A second larger double blind randomised controlled trial compared danazol 200 mg/day with tamoxifen 10 mg/day or placebo. Both danazol and tamoxifen were effective in treating breast pain compared with placebo, but women taking tamoxifen reported fewer side effects. Restricting its use to the luteal phase of the menstrual cycle can reduce the side effects of danazol. In a double blind randomised controlled trial of danazol taken only during the luteal phase compared with placebo, mastalgia was improved by danazol without excess side effects compared with the placebo.

Tamoxifen
Tamoxifen 20 mg/day has been shown to be superior to placebo in one double blind randomised controlled trial, and pain relief was maintained in 72% one year after use. When tamoxifen 10 mg/day was compared with danazol 200 mg/day, tamoxifen was superior to danazol because women reported fewer side effects and more tamoxifen patients (53%) were pain free at one year than in the danazol group (37%).

Giving tamoxifen only in the luteal phase of the menstrual cycle abolished pain in 85% of women, regardless of whether they took 10 mg/day or 20 mg/day. A quarter of the women in the 10 mg group had pain at one year compared with 30% in the 20 mg group; side effects were reported in 21% and 35%, respectively, and included hot flushes and vaginal discharge.

Other hormone based treatments
Progestogens and progesterone have been used orally, topically (applied to the skin of the breast), and vaginally. Compared with placebo oral medroxyprogesterone acetate did not produce any

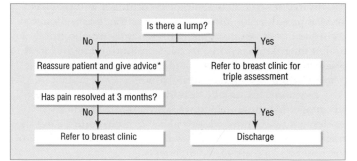

Patient presents to GP with breast pain (*wear supportive well fitting bra, take simple analgesic for pain, regular gentle exercise, low fat diet, cut back on excessive caffeine intake, try agnus castus)

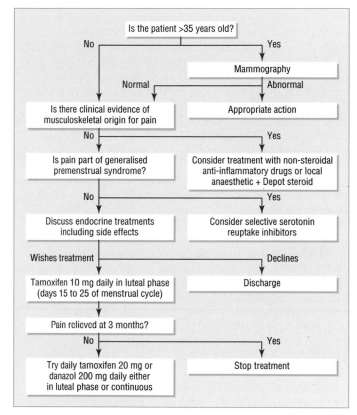

Management of breast pain in breast clinic

Tamoxifen is not currently licensed for breast pain, and there are concerns that long term use in healthy women is associated with an increased risk of deep vein thrombosis and endometrial cancer. These problems, however, are almost exclusively seen in postmenopausal women and although side effects are often reported in premenopausal women, serious adverse events in younger women are uncommon. Studies with tamoxifen gel applied topically to the breast suggest that this may be as effective as oral treatment without the side effects

benefit in a dose of 20 mg/day given during the luteal phase. Topical progesterone produced no benefit in two randomised controlled trials but in a double blind randomised controlled trial of microionised progesterone administered in the luteal phase 65% of treated women and 22% of patients receiving placebo had a 50% reduction in pain.

Gestrinone, a synthetic steroid similar to danazol, has the advantage that the woman does not require additional contraception. Compared with placebo, gestrinone 2.5 mg twice a week produced a greater reduction in pain, but 41% of the women complained of side effects.

Dopamine agonists, such as bromocriptine and lisuride maleate, which inhibit prolactin release, seem effective in reducing breast pain. Although bromocriptine is effective at relieving pain compared with placebo, it is less effective than danazol and up to 80% of women develop side effects including headaches and dizziness. It is thus no longer used to treat breast pain. A placebo controlled trial has shown that lisuride is effective in reducing breast pain.

Non-hormonal treatments

Individual phyto-oestrogens, such as genistein and isoflavins, and soya milk, which is rich in genistein, have been investigated as treatments for breast pain. Only soya milk has been subjected to a double blind randomised controlled study, with cows' milk being used as a control. An improvement in symptoms was noted in 56% of test patients and 10% of controls but the authors reported that non-compliance was a problem. Serum levels of phyto-oestrogens were not raised in some patients who reported a response to treatment, suggesting that they were not actually taking the soya. The major reason for non-compliance was that the soya drink was considered unpalatable.

Agnus castus, a fruit extract, has been subjected to a double blind randomised controlled trial for the treatment of both premenstrual syndrome and mastalgia. Treatment with agnus castus showed an improvement in visual analogue scores and treatment was well tolerated.

Meta-analysis of 10 double blind randomised controlled trials of selective serotonin reuptake inhibitors (SSRIs) used in women with premenstrual symptoms, including four studies that specifically included physical symptoms, showed SSRIs to be more effective than placebo at relieving breast pain. Interestingly, SSRIs did have an effect on fatty acid profiles.

Conclusion

Several treatments are available to treat mastalgia, but there is no single ideal therapy. Reassurance is the mainstay of treatment and is effective. Tamoxifen 10 mg limited to the luteal phase of the menstrual cycle produces the best results with few short term side effects and the lowest recurrence rates of pain at one year but it is not licensed for the treatment of mastalgia. Danazol given in the luteal phase is also effective and limits side effects. For women who have mastalgia as part of premenstrual syndrome, agnus castus or an SSRI are options.

Further studies of more tolerable dietary manipulations are needed. Studies evaluating more palatable soya supplements may be worthwhile. EPO has yet to be shown as an effective agent, and needs to be studied more rigorously, including a "run in" study to exclude women who respond to placebo.

Further reading

- Peters F, Pickardt CR, Zimmerman G, Breckwoldt M. PRL, TSH and thyroid hormones in benign breast disease. *Klinische Wochenschrift* 1981;59:403–7.
- Gateley CA, Maddox PR, Pritchard GA, Sheridan W, Harrison BJ, Pye JK, et al. Plasma fatty acid profiles in benign breast disorders. *Br J Surg* 1992;79:407–9.
- Barros AC, Mottola J, Ruiz CA, Borges MN, Pinotti JA. Reassurance in the treatment of mastalgia. *Breast J* 1999;5:162–5.
- Pashby NH, Mansel RE, Hughes LE, Hanslip J, Preece PE. A clinical trial of evening primrose oil in mastalgia. *Br J Surg* 1981;68:801.
- Boyd NF, McGuire V, Shannon P, Cousins M, Kriukov V, Mahoney L. Effect of a low-fat high-carbohydrate diet on symptoms of clinical mastopathy. *Lancet* 1988;ii:128–32.
- Mishra SK, Sharma AK, Salila M, Srivastava AK, Bal S, Ramesh V. Efficacy of low fat diet in the treatment of benign breast disease. *Nat Med J India* 1994;7:60–62.
- Mansel RE, Wisby JR, Hughes LE. Controlled trial of the antigonadotrophin danazol in painful nodular benign breast disease. *Lancet* 1982:928–31.
- Kontostolis E, Stefanidis K, Navrozoglou I, Lolis D. Comparison of tamoxifen with danazol for treatment of cyclical mastalgia. *Gynecol Endocrinol* 1997;11:393–7.
- O'Brien PM, Abukhalil IE. Randomised controlled trial of the management of premenstrual syndrome and premenstrual mastalgia using luteal phase-only danazol. *Am J Obstet Gynecol* 1999;180:18–23.
- GEMB Group Argentine. Tamoxifen therapy for cyclical mastalgia: dose randomised trial. *Breast* 1997;5:212–13.
- Tamoxifen and venous thromboembolism. Epinet message from department of health. www.doh.gov.uk/cmo/cmo02_04htm
- Maddox PR, Harrison BJ, Horobin JM, Walker K, Mansel RE, Preece PE, et al. A randomised controlled trial of medroxyprogesterone acetate in mastalgia. *Ann R Coll Surg Engl* 1990;72:71–6.
- Peters F. Multicentre study of gestrinone in cyclical breast pain. *Lancet* 1992;339:205–8.
- Kaleli S, Aydin Y, Erel CT, Colgar U. Symptomatic treatment of premenstrual mastalgia in premenopausal women with lisuride maleate: a double blind placebo controlled randomised study. *Fertil Steril* 2001;75:718–23.
- McFayden IJ, Chetty U, Setchell KDR, Zimmer-Nechemias L, Stanley E, Miller WR. A randomized double blind cross over trial of soya protein for the treatment of cyclical breast pain. *Breast* 2000;9:271–6.
- Schellenberg R. Treatment for the premenstrual syndrome with agnus castus fruit extract: prospective randomised controlled study. *BMJ* 2001;322:134–7.
- Halaska M, Raus K, Beles P, Martan A, Paithner KG. Treatment of cyclical mastodynia using an extract of Vitex agnus castus: results of a double blind comparison with a placebo. *Ceska Gynecol* 1998;63:388–92.
- The Cochrane Library, 2002, Issue 14.

4 Breast infection

JM Dixon

Breast infection is now much less common than it used to be. It is seen occasionally in neonates, but it most commonly affects women aged between 18 and 50; in this age group it can be divided into lactational and non-lactational infection. The infection can affect the skin overlying the breast, when it can be a primary event, or it may develop secondary either to a lesion in the skin, such as a sebaceous cyst, or to an underlying skin condition, such as hidradenitis suppurativa.

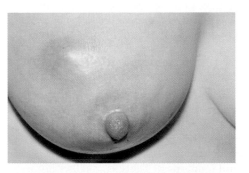

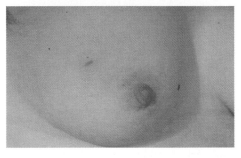

A breast abscess that developed during breast feeding. Before treatment (top), and after mini incision and drainage (bottom)

Organisms responsible for breast infection

Type of breast infection	Organism
Neonatal	*Staphylococcus aureus* (rarely *Escherichia coli*)
Lactating	*S aureus* (rarely *S epidermidis* and streptococci)
Non-lactating	*S aureus*, enterococci, anaerobic streptococci, *Bacteroides* spp
Skin associated	*S aureus*

Treatment

There are four guiding principles in treating breast infection:

- Appropriate antibiotics should be given early to reduce formation of abscesses
- Hospital referral is indicated if the infection does not settle rapidly with one course of antibiotic treatment
- If an abscess is suspected it should be confirmed by ultrasonography, aspiration, or both, before surgical drainage is considered
- Breast cancer should be excluded in patients with an inflammatory lesion that is solid on ultrasonography or on aspiration and that does not settle despite apparently adequate antibiotic treatment.

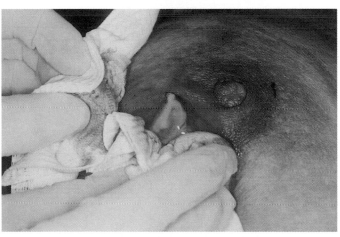

Abscess being drained under local anaesthetic—a small skin incision only is needed

Antibiotics most appropriate for treating breast infections*

Type of breast infection	No allergy to penicillin	Allergy to penicillin
Neonatal, lactating, and skin associated	Flucloxacillin (500 mg four times daily)	Erythromycin (500 mg twice daily)
Non-lactating	Co-amoxiclav (375 mg three times daily)	Combination of erythromycin (500 mg twice daily) with metronidazole (200 mg three times daily)

*Adult doses

All abscesses in the breast can be managed by repeated aspiration or incision and drainage. Ultrasonography is useful to detect pus if this is not obvious clinically. Only a small incision is required to drain a breast abscess adequately. Aspiration is best performed with ultrasound guidance with the abscess cavity being lavaged with local anaesthetic to reduce pain. Incision and drainage, if indicated, can nearly always be performed under local anaesthesia except in children; placement of a drain after incision and drainage is unnecessary. 1% lignocaine containing 1 in 200 000 adrenaline is injected into the skin overlying the abscess. After incision the abscess is irrigated with the same local anaesthetic solution to limit the pain of the procedure.

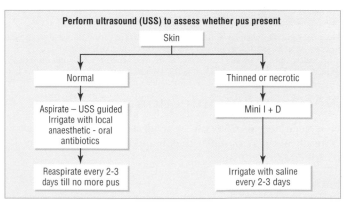

Breast abscesses protocol

Neonatal infection

Neonatal breast infection is most common in the first few weeks of life when the breast bud is enlarged. Although *Staphylococcus aureus* is the usual organism, occasionally infection is due to *Escherichia coli*. If an abscess develops the incision to drain the pus should be placed as peripheral as possible to avoid damaging the breast bud.

Lactating infection

Better maternal and infant hygiene and early treatment with antibiotics have considerably reduced the incidence of abscess formation during lactation. Infection is most commonly seen within the first six weeks of breast feeding, although some women develop it during weaning. Lactating infection presents with pain, swelling, and tenderness. There is usually a history of a cracked nipple or skin abrasion, but this is not the site of entry of organisms. *S aureus* is the most common organism responsible, but *S epidermidis* and streptococci are occasionally isolated. Drainage of milk from the affected segment is often reduced and should be encouraged by continuing breast feeding. Tetracycline, ciprofloxacin, and chloramphenicol should not be used to treat lactating breast infection as they may enter breast milk and can harm the baby.

If the infection does not settle after one course of flucloxacillin and no pus is detected on ultrasonography or obtained on aspiration and if cytology indicates the lesion is infective or inflammatory, the antibiotic should be changed to co-amoxiclav to cover other possible pathogens. If inflammation or an associated mass lesion still persists, further investigation is required to exclude an underlying carcinoma. Established abscesses should be treated by either repeated aspiration—every two to three days until no more pus is aspirated—or incision and drainage. Women who want to continue breast feeding should be encouraged to do so.

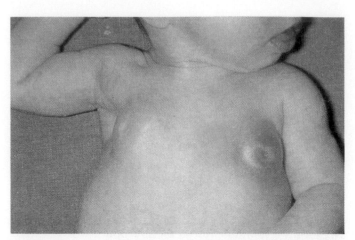

Neonatal breast abscess (reproduced with permission from RE Mansel)

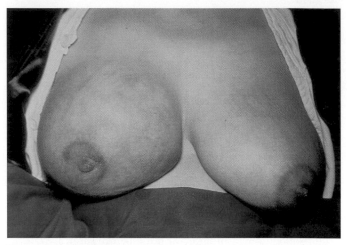

Puerperal mastitis of right breast. Note erythema, oedema, and obvious signs of inflammation, especially medially

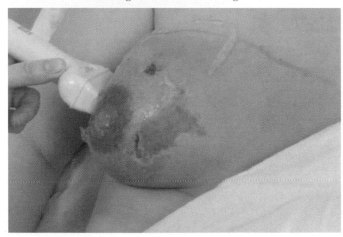

Hospital referral was delayed in this patient with a lactating breast abscess. Skin necrosis developed due to pressure in the abscess and infection.
Ultrasonography showed a large central abscess, which resolved after multiple aspirations. The resulting skin loss and asymmetry required subsequent surgery

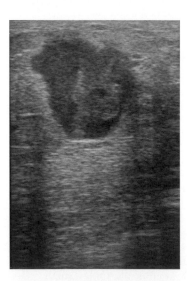

Ultrasound picture of lactating breast abscess

Non-lactating infection

Non-lactating infections can be separated into those that occur centrally in the periareolar region and those that affect the peripheral breast tissue.

Periareolar infection

Periareolar infection is most commonly seen in young women (mean age 32). Histologically, there is active inflammation around non-dilated subareolar breast ducts—a condition that is called periductal mastitis. This condition has been confused

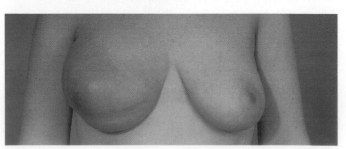

Inflammatory carcinoma of right breast. Note erythema and peau d'orange

with and called duct ectasia, but duct ectasia is a separate condition affecting older women and is characterised by subareolar duct dilatation and less pronounced and less active periductal inflammation. Current evidence suggests that smoking is an important factor in the aetiology of periductal mastitis but not in duct ectasia: about 90% of women who get periductal mastitis or its complications smoke cigarettes compared with 38% of the same age group in the general population. Substances in cigarette smoke may either directly or indirectly damage the wall of the subareolar breast ducts. Aerobic or anaerobic organisms then infect the damaged tissues. Initial presentation may be with periareolar inflammation (with or without an associated mass) or with an established abscess. Associated features include central breast pain, nipple retraction at the site of the diseased duct, and nipple discharge.

Treatment

A periareolar inflammatory mass should be treated with a course of appropriate antibiotics and investigated by ultrasonography; any abscess found should be managed by aspiration or incision and drainage. If the mass is solid on ultrasonography or inflammation does not resolve after appropriate treatment, care should be taken to exclude an underlying neoplasm. Abscesses associated with periductal mastitis commonly recur because treatment by aspiration or incision does not remove the underlying diseased duct. Up to a third of patients develop a mammary duct fistula after drainage of a non-lactating periareolar abscess. Recurrent episodes of periareolar sepsis should be treated by excision of diseased ducts under antibiotic cover by an experienced breast surgeon.

Mammary duct fistula

A mammary duct fistula is a communication between the skin, usually in the periareolar region, and a major subareolar breast duct. A fistula can develop after incision and drainage of a non-lactating abscess, it can follow spontaneous discharge of a periareolar inflammatory mass, or it can result from biopsy of a periductal inflammatory mass.

Treatment

Treatment is by excision of the fistula and diseased duct or ducts under antibiotic cover. Recurrence is common after surgery, and the lowest rates of recurrence and best cosmetic results tend to be achieved in specialist breast units.

Peripheral non-lactating breast abscesses

These are less common than periareolar abscesses and can be associated with an underlying condition such as diabetes, rheumatoid arthritis, steroid treatment, granulomatous lobular mastitis, and trauma. Infection associated with granulomatous

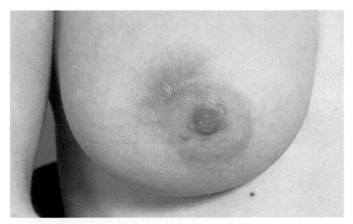

Periareolar inflammation due to periductal mastitis. Minor degree of nipple retraction is present at the site of the affected duct

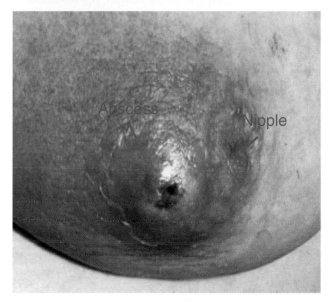

Non-lactating breast abscess due to periductal mastitis. Arrows point to inverted nipple and abscess

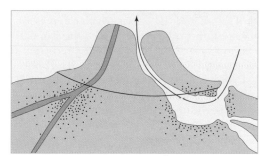

Mammary duct fistula with arrow showing path of fistula probe. Dots around duct on left represent periductal mastitis, a precursor of a fistula

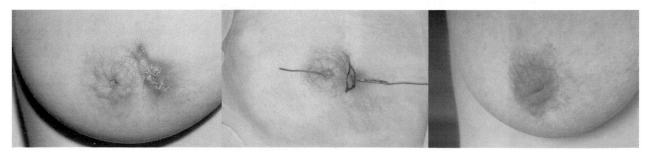

Mammary duct fistula. Left: external opening at areola margin, entire nipple is inverted; middle: probe passed through opening of fistula and emerging from affected duct; right: after excision of fistula and affected duct and primary wound closure under antibiotic cover. Operation performed through a circumareolar incision, which gives excellent cosmetic results

lobular mastitis can be a particular problem. This condition affects young parous women, who may develop large areas of infection with multiple simultaneous peripheral abscesses. One study isolated corynebacteria from such lesions, but as antibiotics effective against these organisms do not lead to rapid resolution of disease, corynebacteria do not therefore appear aetiological in this condition. There is a strong tendency for this condition to persist and recur after surgery. Large incisions and extensive surgery should therefore be avoided. Steroids have been tried but with limited success and are not recommended. Peripheral breast abscesses should be treated by recurrent aspiration or incision and drainage.

Rarely subareolar or peripheral non-lactating infection can occur as a consequence of infection of an area of comedo necrosis associated with ductal carcinoma in situ. After antibiotic treatment or aspiration of pus, these areas can resolve completely and leave no residual mass. For this reason, all patients aged >35 should have a mammogram after resolution of an infective episode.

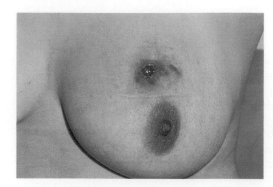

Granulomatous lobular mastitis of left breast

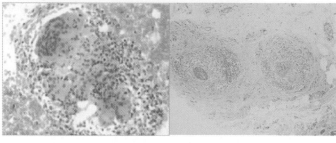

Granulomata seen in fine needle aspirate (left) and in a core biopsy sample from granulomatous lobular mastitis

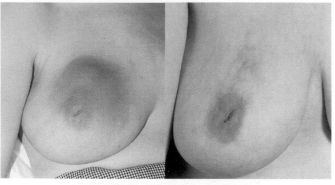

Peripheral breast abscess before management (left) and after recurrent aspiration and oral antibiotics (right)

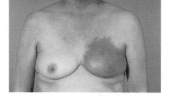

Cellulitis of left breast that occurred 18 months after left wide local excision and radiotherapy

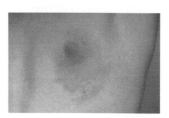

Cellulitis of left breast of an adolescent man

Skin associated infection

Primary infection of the skin of the breast, which can present as cellulitis or an abscess, most commonly affects the skin of the lower half of the breast. These infections are often recurrent in women who are overweight, have large breasts, or have poor personal hygiene. Cellulitis most commonly affects the skin of the breast after surgery or radiotherapy. *S aureus* is the usual causative organism, though fungal infections have been reported. Cellulitis in the male breast is uncommon but is seen in the neonatal and pubertal periods.

Treatment of acute bacterial infection is with antibiotics and drainage or aspiration of abscesses. Women with recurrent infections should be advised about weight reduction and keeping the area as clean and dry as possible (this includes careful washing of the area up to twice a day, using a hair dryer to dry the skin, avoiding skin creams and talcum powder, and wearing either a cotton bra or a cotton T shirt or vest worn inside the bra).

Sebaceous cysts are common in the skin of the breast and may become infected. Some recurrent infections in the inframammary fold are due to hidradenitis suppurativa. In this condition, infection should be controlled with appropriate antibiotics and drainage of any pus (the same organisms are found in hidradenitis as in non-lactating infection). Excision of the affected skin is effective at stopping further infection in about half of patients; the remainder go on to have further episodes of infection despite surgery.

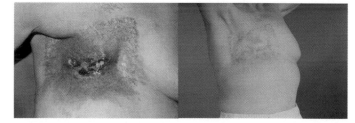

Cellulitis of right breast 10 years after mastectomy, insertion of prosthesis, and mastectomy (left). Areas of ulceration are due to erosion of prosthesis through the skin (rarely seen with current radiotherapy techniques). Same patient (right) after wound settled and healed with treatment with co-amoxiclav

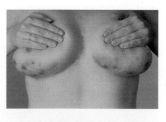

Hidradenitis suppurativa, causing recurrent skin infection of lower half of breast

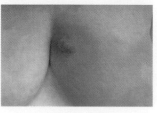

Infected sebaceous cyst

Other infections and inflammatory conditions

Tuberculosis of the breast is now rare and can be primary or, more commonly, secondary. Clues to its diagnosis include the presence of a breast or axillary sinus in up to half of patients. The commonest presentation of tuberculosis nowadays is with an abscess resulting from infection of a tuberculous cavity by an acute pyogenic organism such as *S aureus*. An open biopsy is often required to establish the diagnosis. Treatment is by a combination of surgery and antituberculous chemotherapy.

Syphilis, actinomycosis, and mycotic, helminthic, and viral infections occasionally affect the breast but are rare. Infection with *Candida albicans* has been implicated in causing deep breast pain after breast feeding. The evidence for this association is extremely weak and does not justify the use of fluconazole in these women.

Nipple rings can cause problems with recurrent infection, particularly in smokers. Rarely, excision of the nipple areolar complex is required to control ongoing infection. The nipple can become irritated from running (jogger's nipple) or regular trauma (tassle dancer's nipple). Pilonidial abscesses affecting the nipple have been reported in hairdressers and sheep shearers. Rarely, spontaneous infarction, also known as primary gangrene of the breast, occurs. Treatment is debridement of dead and infected tissue.

Lymphocytic lobulitis

Also known as sclerosing lymphocytic lobulitis, lymphocytic lobulitis is associated in some patients with autoimmune disorders. A similar condition occurs in people with diabetes and is known as diabetic mastopathy or lymphocytic mastitis. These conditions present as a mass that can resemble malignancy. They are characterised histologically by intense fibrosis associated with lymphocytic infiltration around lobules and epithelioid fibroblasts in the stroma. No specific treatment is required once the diagnosis is established. Diagnosis is usually possible on core biopsy.

Factitial disease

Artefactual or factitial diseases are created by the patient, often through complicated or repetitive actions. Such patients may undergo many investigations and operations before the nature of the disease is recognised. The diagnosis is difficult to establish but should be considered when the clinical situation does not conform to common appearances or pathological processes. There is often a history of multiple visits to both general practitioner and hospital with various symptoms. Psychiatric referral may help in establishing the diagnosis but there is no recognised effective therapy.

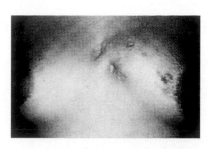

Tuberculosis of left breast with multiple sinuses

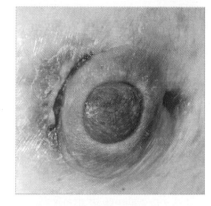

Recurrent persistent infection, despite repeated drainage. Infection started after insertion of a nipple ring

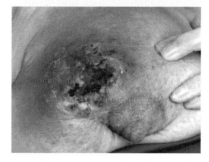

Spontaneous infarction, also known as primary gangrene of the breast. In this patient, who had diabetes, the dead tissue was excised on two occasions before the wound eventually healed

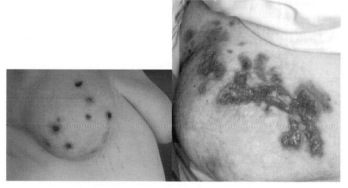

Factitial disease is caused by repetitive trauma. When covered by an occlusive dressing, the wounds in both patients healed. Patient on the right had a history of seeking frequent medical attention

Further reading

- Bundred NJ. The aetiology of periductal mastitis. *Breast* 1993;2:1–2.
- Bundred NJ, Dixon JM, Lumsden AB, Radford D, Hood J, Miles RS, et al. Are the lesions of duct ectasia sterile? *Br J Surg* 1985;72:844–5.
- Dixon JM. Repeated aspiration of breast abscesses in lactating women. *Br Med J* 1988;297:1517–18.
- Dixon JM, RaviSekar O, Chetty O, Anderson TJ. Periductal mastitis and duct ectasia: different conditions with different aetiologies. *Br J Surg* 1996;83:820–22.
- Hughes LE, Mansel RE, Webster DJT. *Benign disorders and diseases of the breast: concepts and clinical management.* 2nd ed. London: Saunders, 2000.
- Dixon JM, Bundred NJ. Management of disorders of the ductal system. In: Harris JR, Lippman ME, Morrow M, Hellman S, eds. *Diseases of the breast.* Philadelphia: Lippincott Williams and Wilkins, 2004:47–56.
- Taylor GB, Paviour SD, Musaad S, Jones WO, Holland DJ. A clinicopathological review of 34 cases of inflammatory breast disease showing an association between corynebacteria infection and granulomatous mastitis. *Pathology* 2003;35:109–19.

5 Breast cancer—epidemiology, risk factors, and genetics

K McPherson, CM Steel, JM Dixon

With over a million new cases in the world each year, breast cancer is the most common malignancy in women and comprises 18% of all female cancers. Age standardised incidence and mortality in the United Kingdom are among the highest in the world. The incidence rates are about 3 per 1000 for 50 year olds, and the disease is the single most common cause of death among women aged 40–50, accounting for a fifth of all deaths in this age group. There are more than 13 000 deaths each year, and the incidence is increasing particularly among women aged 50–64, probably because of breast screening in this age group. Age standardised incidence increased by 18% between 1990 and 1999 and will increase by over 20% between 2000 and 2010.

Of every 1000 women aged 50, two will recently have had breast cancer diagnosed and about 15 will have had a diagnosis made before the age of 50, giving a prevalence of nearly 2%. In the European Union one million women are alive with breast cancer.

Worldwide incidence of cancers in women

Site of cancer	1000s of cases	% of total
Breast	572	18
Cervix	466	15
Colon and rectum	286	9
Stomach	261	8
Endometrium	149	5
Lung	147	5
Ovary	138	4
Mouth and pharynx	121	4
Oesophagus	108	4
Lymphoid tissue	98	3

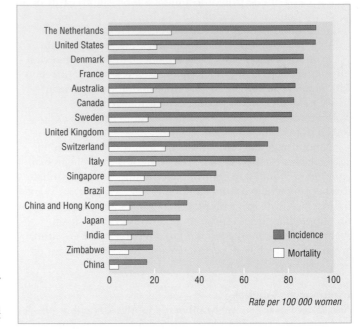

Age standardised world incidence of and mortality from breast cancer in different countries. Adapted from Cancer Stats, Cancer Research UK, 2003

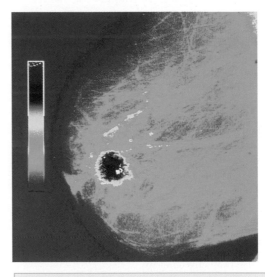

Computer enhanced mammogram of a breast cancer

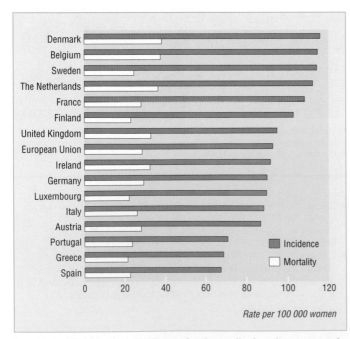

Age standardised European incidence of and mortality from breast cancer in different countries. Adapted from Cancer Stats, Cancer Research UK, 2003

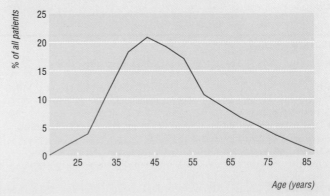

Percentage of all deaths in women attributable to breast cancer

Risk factors for breast cancer

Age

The incidence of breast cancer increases with age, doubling about every 10 years until the menopause, when the rate of increase slows dramatically. Compared with lung cancer, the incidence of breast cancer is higher at younger ages. In some countries there is a flattening of the age-incidence curve after the menopause.

Risk of developing breast cancer by age, England, 1996*

Risk up to:

25 years—1 in 15 000	70 years—1 in 15
30 years—1 in 1900	80 years—1 in 11
40 years—1 in 200	85 years—1 in 10
50 years—1 in 50	Lifetime risk (all ages)—1 in 9
60 years—1 in 23	

*Adapted from CancerStats—Breast Cancer UK 2003

Geographical variation

Age adjusted incidence and mortality for breast cancer varies by up to a factor of five between countries. The difference between Far Eastern and Western countries is diminishing but is still about fivefold. In migrants from Japan to Hawaii the rates of breast cancer assume the rate in the host country within one or two generations, indicating that environmental factors are of greater importance than genetic factors.

Age at menarche and menopause

Women who start menstruating early in life or who have a late menopause have an increased risk of developing breast cancer. Women who have a natural menopause after the age of 55 are twice as likely to develop breast cancer as women who experience the menopause before the age of 45. At one extreme, women who undergo bilateral oophorectomy before the age of 35 have only 40% of the risk of breast cancer in women who have a natural menopause.

Age at first pregnancy

Nulliparity and late age at first birth both increase the lifetime incidence of breast cancer. The risk of breast cancer in women who have their first child after the age of 30 is about twice that of women who have their first child before the age of 20. The highest risk group is those who have a first child after the age of 35; these women seem to be at even higher risk than nulliparous women. An early age at birth of a second child further reduces the risk of breast cancer.

Family history

Up to 10% of breast cancer in Western countries is due to strong genetic predisposition. Susceptibility to breast cancer is generally inherited as an autosomal dominant with limited penetrance. This means that it can be transmitted through either sex and that some family members may transmit the abnormal gene without developing cancer themselves. It is not yet known how many breast cancer genes there are. Two such genes, BRCA1 and BRCA2, which are located on the long arms of chromosomes 17 and 13, respectively, have been identified and account for a substantial proportion of families that are considered to be very high risk—that is, those with four or more breast cancers among close relatives. Both genes are large and mutations can occur at almost any position so that molecular screening to detect mutation for the first time in an affected individual or family is technically demanding.

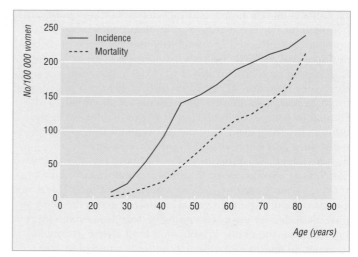

Age specific incidence and mortality for breast cancer in the United Kingdom

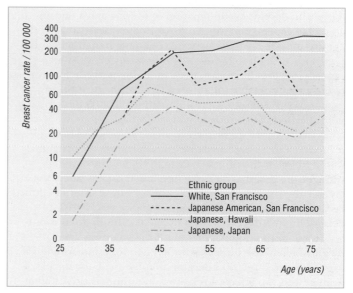

Annual incidence of breast cancer in Japanese women in Japan, Hawaii, and San Francisco, and in white women from San Francisco

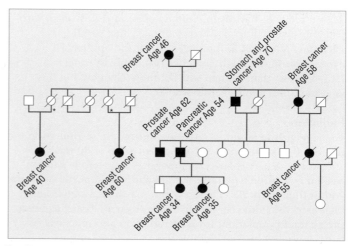

Family tree of family with genetically inherited breast cancer

Certain mutations occur at high frequency in defined populations. For instance, some 2% of Ashkenazim Jewish women carry BRCA1 185 del AG (deletion of two base pairs in position 185), BRCA1 5382 ins C (insertion of an extra base pair at position 5382), or BRCA 6174 del T (deletion of a single base pair at position 6174), while BRCA2 999 del 5 (deletion of five base pairs at position 999) accounts for about half of all familial breast cancer in Iceland. Inherited mutations in two other genes, p53 and PTEN, are associated with familial syndromes (Li-Fraumeni and Cowden's, respectively) that include a high risk of breast cancer but both are rare. A few families are also described in which multiple cases of breast cancer are attributed to mutations in ATM or Chk2. There are almost certainly other (as yet unidentified) genes that increase the risk of disease by only a moderate degree—perhaps three or four times the general population level. These are unlikely to generate multi-case families, but they are probably rather common and therefore account for a substantial part of the overall genetic contribution to breast cancer.

Many families affected by breast cancer show an excess of ovarian, colon, prostatic, and other cancers attributable to the same inherited mutation. Patients with bilateral breast cancer, those who develop a combination of breast cancer and another epithelial cancer, and women who get the disease at an early age are most likely to be carrying a genetic mutation that has predisposed them to developing breast cancer. Most breast cancers that are due to a genetic mutation occur before the age of 65, and a woman with a strong family history of breast cancer of early onset who is still unaffected at 65 has probably not inherited the genetic mutation.

A woman's risk of breast cancer is two or more times greater if she has a first degree relative (mother, sister, or daughter) who developed the disease before the age of 50; and the younger the relative when she developed breast cancer the greater the risk. For example, a woman whose sister developed breast cancer aged 30–39 has a cumulative risk of 10% of developing the disease herself by age 65, but that risk is only 5% (close to the population risk) if the sister was aged 50–54 at diagnosis. The risk increases by between four and six times if two first degree relatives develop the disease. For example, a woman with two affected relatives, one who was aged <50 at diagnosis, has a 25% chance of developing breast cancer by the age of 65.

Previous benign breast disease

Women with severe atypical epithelial hyperplasia have four to five times the risk of developing breast cancer than women who do not have any proliferative changes in their breasts. Women with this change and a family history of breast cancer (first degree relative) have a ninefold increase in risk. Women with palpable cysts, complex fibroadenomas, duct papillomas, sclerosing adenosis, and moderate or florid epithelial hyperplasia have a slightly higher risk of breast cancer (1.5–3 times) than women without these changes, but this increase is not clinically important.

Radiation

Teenage girls exposed to radiation during the second world war had double the risk of developing cancer up to 30 years afterwards. A particular contemporary risk group is women treated by mantle type radiotherapy for lymphoma as teenagers and in their early 20s. These women may have a significantly increased risk, and require screening from an earlier age than the general population. Ionising radiation also increases risk later in life but by considerably less.

Familial breast cancer

Criteria for identifying women at substantial increased risk

The following categories identify women who have three or more times the population risk of developing breast cancer

A woman who has:
  One first degree* relative with bilateral breast cancer or breast and ovarian cancer *or*
  One first degree relative with breast cancer diagnosed under the age of 40 or one first degree male relative with breast cancer diagnosed at any age *or*
  Two first or second degree relatives with breast cancer diagnosed under the age of 60 or ovarian cancer at any age on the same side of the family *or*
  Three first or second degree relatives with breast and ovarian cancer on the same side of the family

Criteria for identifying women at very high risk in whom gene testing might be appropriate

Families with four or more relatives affected with either breast or ovarian cancer in three generations and one alive affected individual

*First degree relative is mother, sister, or daughter; second degree female relative is grandmother, granddaughter, aunt, or niece

Established and probable risk factors for breast cancer

Factor	Relative risk	High risk group
Age	>10	Elderly
Geographical location	5	Developed country
Age at menarche	3	Before age 11
Age at menopause	2	After age 54
Age at 1st full pregnancy	3	First child in early 40s
Family history	≥2	Breast cancer in first degree relative when young
Previous benign disease	4–5	Atypical hyperplasia
Cancer in other breast	>4	
Socioeconomic group	2	Groups I and II
Diet	1.5	High intake of saturated fat
Premenopausal	0.7	Body mass index >35
Postmenopausal	2	Body mass index >35
Alcohol consumption	1.3	Excessive intake
Exposure to ionising radiation	3	Abnormal exposure in young females > age 10
Taking exogenous hormones:		
Oral contraceptives	1.24	Current use
Combined hormone replacement therapy	2.3	Use for ≥10 years
Unopposed oestrogen	1.3	Use for ≥10 years
Diethylstilbestrol	2	Use during pregnancy

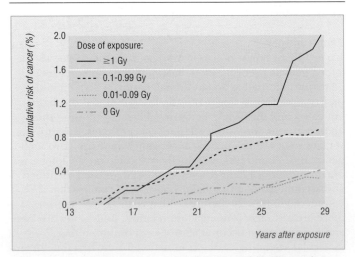

Cumulative risk of breast cancer in women who were aged 10–19 years when they were exposed to radiation from atomic bombs during the second world war

Lifestyle

Hormone replacement therapy

Among current users of hormone replacement therapy (HRT) and those who stopped using it one to four years before the relative risk of having breast cancer increases by a factor of 1.023 (1.011 to 1.036 95% CI) for each year of use. This increase is consistent with the effect of a delay in menopause because the relative risk of breast cancer increases in women who have never used HRT by a factor of 1.028 (1.021 to 1.034) for each year delay in natural menopause. The risk of breast cancer is higher with combined oestrogen and progestogen, amounting to a doubling of risk after five years of use. This risk seems independent of the dose of oestrogen, type of oestrogen, and mode of delivery (oral or transdermal). The same is true for progestogen content. Whether progestogen only treatment increases risk is not clear. Vaginal oestrogen does not seem to increase the risk of breast cancer.

The effect of HRT on risk is concentrated among current users. Oestrogen supplements alone among women without a uterus do not affect the risk of breast cancer and possibly lower it, although many such women will also have had a bilateral oophorectomy, which lowers risk. HRT increases breast density and thus reduces both the sensitivity and specificity of breast screening. Tibolone, a gonadomimetic agent, is almost as effective as combined HRT in relieving menopausal symptoms but does not seem to have the same effect as combined HRT in increasing breast density. It can be used only in women who have stopped menstruating. In the million women study it seemed to increase the risk of developing breast cancer, but the increase was less than that associated with combined HRT.

Early studies suggested that the type and stage of breast cancer that women developed on HRT was more favourable. Data from the women's health initiative study, however, have shown that the breast cancers diagnosed in women taking HRT were larger and more likely to be node positive.

Effects of HRT on breast screening

In 103 770 screened women aged 50–69 years:

- Sensitivity
  64.3% (57–72 95% CI) in users
  79.8% (76–84) in non-users
- False negative rate
  Odds ratio 1.60 (1.04–2.21 95% CI) for users
- Specificity
  0.6% lower in users, P < 0.002
- False positive rate
  Odds ratio 1.12 (1.05 to 1.19) P = 0.0004

From Kavanagh AM et al. *Lancet* 2000;355:270–4

Weight

Obesity is associated with a twofold increase in the risk of breast cancer in postmenopausal women, whereas before the menopause it is associated with a slightly reduced incidence.

Height

There has been a reported increase in risk of breast cancer of 5% for every 5 cm increase in height in premenopausal women and 10% for each 5 cm in postmenopausal women.

Breast feeding

Each year that a woman breast feeds reduces her risk by about 4%.

Diet

Although there is a correlation between the incidence of breast cancer and dietary fat intake at a population level, the true

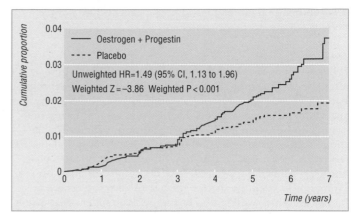

Effect of HRT on risk of breast cancer. Data from women's health institute (WHI) study, a randomised trial comparing combined HRT with placebo. Data are based on women who were taking HRT. Adapted from *JAMA* 2003; 289:3243–53

Combined HRT and breast cancer stage from women's health initiative (WHI) study

- Mean 5.2 years' follow up
- Breast cancers on HRT were larger: 1.7 cm *v* 1.5, P = 0.04
- Patients on HRT more likely to be node positive: 25.4% *v* 16.0%, P = 0.04

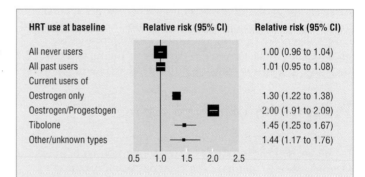

Risk of breast cancer related to type of HRT. Adapted from the Million Women Study, *Lancet* 2003;362:419–27

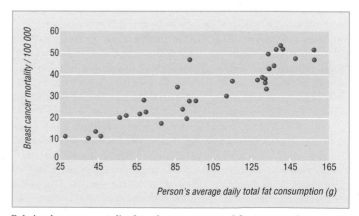

Relation between mortality from breast cancer and fat consumption

relation between fat intake and breast cancer does not seem to be particularly strong or consistent.

Oral contraceptives
While women are taking oral contraceptives and for 10 years after they stop, there is a small increase in the risk of developing breast cancer. There is no significantly increased risk 10 or more years after stopping. Cancers diagnosed in women taking oral contraceptives seem less likely to be advanced clinically than those diagnosed in women who have never done so (relative risk 0.88 (% CI 0.81–0.95)). Duration of use, age at first use, dose, and type of hormone seem to have no significant effect on risk. Women who begin use before the age of 20 seem to have a higher risk than women who begin use at an older age, possibly because of higher rates of proliferation among nulliparous users. This higher risk "applies" at an age when the incidence of breast cancer is low.

Alcohol intake
Several studies have shown a link between alcohol consumption and incidence of breast cancer, but the association may be with other dietary factors rather than with alcohol.

Smoking
Most studies find no excess of breast cancers in smokers that cannot be accounted for by confounding with alcohol. There are some data linking passive smoking with risk, the most plausible explanation being an inadequate adjustment in these studies for confounding. It is unlikely that smoking has an important aetiological role in breast cancer.

Abortion
An overview of 53 studies shows no effect of either spontaneous or induced abortion on risk, when abortion history is recorded before diagnosis. In studies in which abortion history is obtained after a diagnosis of breast cancer the relative risk is 1.1 for induced abortion, which is attributable to bias in reporting.

Prevention of breast cancer

Screening as currently practiced can reduce mortality but not incidence and is cost effective only among women in whom breast cancer is common (>2/1000 per year). Advances in treatment—hormonal and cytotoxic—and better delivery of care have also produced considerable survival benefits. A greater appreciation of factors important in the aetiology of breast cancer would raise the possibility of disease prevention.

Hormonal control
One promising avenue for primary prevention is influencing the hormonal milieu of women at risk. During trials of tamoxifen, which is now known to be a selective oestrogen receptor modulator (SERM), used as an adjuvant treatment for breast cancer, the number of contralateral breast cancers was smaller than expected, suggesting that this drug might have a role in preventing breast cancer. Studies comparing tamoxifen with placebo in women at high risk of breast cancer have been reported and show varied results.

The NSABP study randomised 3338 women with a risk equal to that of a 60 year old woman and showed a 47% reduction in the risk of invasive breast cancer and a 50% reduction in the rate of non-invasive breast cancer in women taking tamoxifen. Benefits of tamoxifen were observed in all age groups. Tamoxifen also reduced the overall incidence of osteoporotic fractures of the hip, spine, and radius by 19% but increased the relative risk of endometrial cancer by 2.5. More women over 50 in the

Relative risk of breast cancer in relation to use of oral contraceptives

	Relative risk (95% CI)
Never used/>10 years since stopped use	1.0
Current user	1.24 (0.96 to 1.05)
1–5 years since stopped use	1.16 (1.08 to 1.23)
5–9 years since stopped use	1.07 (1.02 to 1.13)

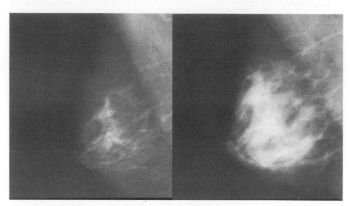

Mammograms before (left) and after (right) three years of hormone replacement therapy showing increase in density caused by treatment

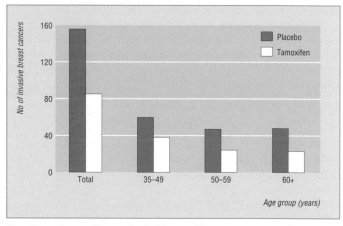

The effect of tamoxifen on the incidence of breast cancer according to age (Data from the NSABP prevention study)

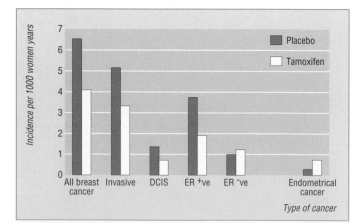

Overview of prevention studies showing incidence of cancer in four tamoxifen prevention trials. DCIS = ductal in situ carcinoma, ER = oestrogen receptor. Adapted from Cuzick J et al, *Lancet* 2003;361:296–300

tamoxifen group developed more deep venous thromboses, pulmonary emboli, and strokes. An overview of all trials showed a 48% reduction in the incidence of tumours positive for oestrogen receptor and no effect on tumours negative for oestrogen receptor, which represents a 38% reduction overall.

Raloxifene, another SERM, which lacks direct endometrial stimulation, has been evaluated in a population of 10 355 postmenopausal women being treated for osteoporosis and was associated with a 54% decrease in the number of breast cancers. Raloxifene also shows a selective effect on breast cancers positive for oestrogen receptor, while seeming to have fewer side effects. Aromatase inhibitors in one adjuvant study reduced the risk of contralateral breast cancers to a greater degree than tamoxifen. They may also prevent tumours negative for oestrogen receptor. These agents reduce oestrogen production and increase bone fractures; clinical trials of their use as preventive agents are in progress.

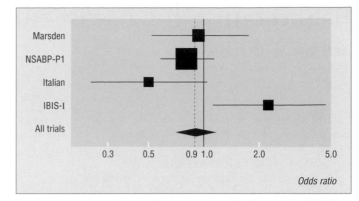

Death from any cause in tamoxifen prevention trials. Error bars = 95% CI

Dietary intervention

If specific dietary factors are found to be associated with an increased risk of breast cancer dietary intervention will be possible. However, reduction of dietary intake of such a factor in whole communities may well be difficult to achieve without major social and cultural changes. An increase in weight of >10–20 kg from the weight at age 18 seems to be associated with an increased risk.

Other preventive agents

Retinoids affect the growth and differentiation of epithelial cells, and experiments suggest that they may have a role in preventing breast cancer. A study of 2972 women with breast cancer randomly allocated to fenretinide or no treatment found no significant difference in contralateral breast cancer between the two groups. There was a significant interaction with treatment and menopausal status with a beneficial effect being seen in premenopausal women (adjusted hazard ratio 0.66, 95% confidence interval 0.14 to 1.07) and an opposite trend in postmenopausal women. Prolonged follow up has confirmed a benefit of fenretinide in younger premenopausal women.

Aspirin and other non-steroidal anti-inflammatory agents taken for long periods are associated with a decrease in the rate of development of breast cancer. Aspirin may operate through effects on oestrogen synthesis and preferentially reduce development of hormone receptor positive breast cancer. One review reported hazard rates of 0.7 for case-control studies and 0.79 for cohort studies. It is thought the effect of aspirin may be mediated through its effects on COX 2 (cyclo-oxygenase-2) inhibitors rather than a COX 1 inhibitor. Selective COX 2 inhibitors such as celecoxib are currently being investigated in a series of studies in different settings.

Selenium is another possible cancer preventing agent.

Further reading

- Bilimoria M, Morrow M. The woman at increased risk for breast cancer: evaluation and management strategies. *Cancer J Clin* 1995;45:263–78.
- Brinton LA, Devesa SS. Etiology and pathogenesis of breast cancer: incidence, demographics and environmental factors. In: Harris JR, Lippman ME, Morrow M, Hellman S, eds. *Diseases of the breast*. Philadelphia: Lippincott–Raven, 1996;159–68.
- Collaborative Group on Hormonal Factors in Breast Cancer. Breast cancer and hormonal contraceptives: collaborative reanalysis of individual data on 53 297 women with breast cancer and 100 239 women without breast cancer from 54 epidemiological studies. *Lancet* 1996;347:1713–27.
- Collaborative Group on Hormonal Factors in Breast Cancer. Breast cancer and hormone replacement therapy: collaborative reanalysis of data from 51 epidemiological studies of 52 705 women with breast cancer and 108 411 without breast cancer. *Lancet* 1997;350:1047–59.
- Collaborative Group on Hormonal Factors in Breast Cancer. Breast cancer and abortion: collaborative reanalysis of data from 53 epidemiological studies, including 83 000 women with breast cancer from 16 countries. *Lancet* 2004;363:1007–16.
- Cuzick J, Powles T, Veronesi U, Forbes J, Edwards R, Ashley S, et al. Overview of the main outcomes in breast cancer prevention trials. *Lancet* 2003;361:296–300.
- Jordan VC, Glusman JE, Eckert S, et al. Raloxifene reduces incident primary breast cancers: integrated data from multicenter double blind placebo controlled, randomised trials in postmenopausal women. *Breast Cancer Res Treat* 1998;50:227.
- Key TJ, Allen NE, Spencer EA. Nutrition and breast cancer. *Breast* 2003;12:412–16.
- Lahmann PH, Hoffmann K, Allen N, van Gils CH, Khaw KT, Tehard B, et al. Body size and breast cancer risk: findings from a European Prospective Investigation into Cancer and Nutrition (EPIC). *Int J Cancer* 2004;111;762–71.
- Million Women Study Collaborators. Breast cancer and hormone-replacement therapy in the Million Women Study. *Lancet* 2003;362:419–27.
- Terry MB, Gammon MD, Zhang FF, Tawfik H, Teitelbaum SL, Britton JA, et al. Association of frequency and duration of aspirin use and hormone receptor status with breast cancer risk. *JAMA* 2004;291;2433–40.
- Writing Group for Women's Health Initiative Investigators. Risks and benefits of estrogen and progestin in healthy postmenopausal women: principle results from the women's health initiative randomised controlled trial. *JAMA* 2002;288:321–33.

6 Screening for breast cancer

ARM Wilson, RD Macmillan, J Patnick

Lack of knowledge of the pathogenesis of breast cancer means that primary prevention is currently a distant prospect for most women. Early detection represents an alternative approach for reducing mortality from this disease.

Screening can be targeted at populations at risk (for example, women aged ≥50) and high risk groups (for example, younger women with a significant genetic risk). There is no evidence that clinical examination or teaching self examination of the breast are effective tools for early detection.

> **The aim of screening is to reduce morbidity and mortality from breast cancer by detecting it early and treating it when it is small and before it has had the chance to spread**

Screening tests should be simple to apply, cheap, easy to perform, easy and unambiguous to interpret, and identify those with disease and exclude those without. Film screen mammography requires high technology equipment, special film and dedicated processing, highly trained staff to perform the examinations, and highly trained readers to interpret the films. Mammography is at present the best screening tool available and was the first screening method for any malignancy that has been shown to be of value in randomised trials. The potential benefits of digital mammography remain to be evaluated. There is some evidence that ultrasonography of the mammographic dense breast can improve sensitivity. Magnetic resonance imaging seems to be valuable in screening younger high risk groups.

Organisation of population screening

- Accurate population lists
- Encouragement by general practitioners to attend
- Clear screening protocols
- Agreed patterns of referral
- Well trained multidisciplinary assessment team
- Built in quality assurance
- Continual audit and education

Population screening

Effect on mortality
Randomised controlled trials have shown that screening by mammography can significantly reduce absolute mortality from breast cancer by up to 40% in those who attend. The benefit is greatest in women aged 50–70. Published data from the combined Swedish trials show an overall significant reduction in mortality from breast cancer of 21% during 15 years of follow up in women aged 40–74, with the most benefit seen in women aged 55–69 (30%).

Acceptance, quality assurance, and monitoring
Over 70% of the target population must participate if screening is to reduce mortality significantly, and the cost per life year saved rises if fewer participate. To achieve optimal participation accurate lists of names, ages, and current addresses are required. Factors affecting attendance for screening include the level of encouragement by general practitioners, knowledge about the disease and the screening programme, and the views and experiences of family and friends. Screening programmes must include both the initial screening process and the assessment of abnormalities detected by screening, and have clearly defined treatment pathways when these are necessary.

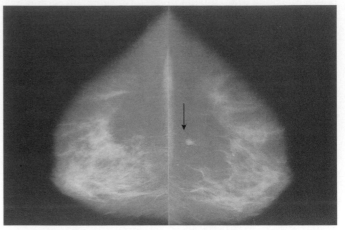

Typical features of small carcinoma (arrow) found on screening mammography, Adapted from Cancer Stats, Cancer Research UK, 2003

Detection of breast cancer after an initial screening in women aged 50–70

	No of women
Initial screen	10 000
Recall for assessment	500–700
Surgical biopsy	<100
Breast cancer detected	60–70

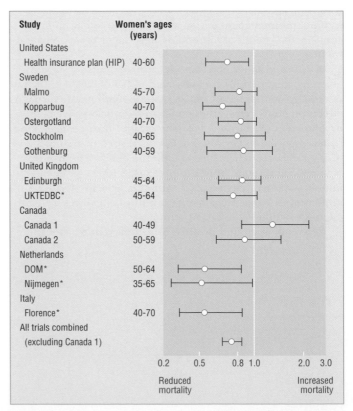

Summary of 7–12 year mortality data from randomised and case-control (*) studies of breast cancer screening. Points and lines represent absolute change in mortality and confidence interval

Standards must be set to ensure that targets for mortality reduction are likely to be achieved and that there is quality assurance at each stage of the screening process. Multidisciplinary teams experienced in the management of breast disease should carry out screening and assessment. Specific training and regular education programmes related to screening should be mandatory for all professionals involved, and regular audit and review of individual and programme results and performance is necessary.

Age range

Current data indicate that absolute reduction in mortality is greatest in women aged 55–69 (30%). A smaller reduction in mortality of 20% could be achieved in younger women (40–54), but screening is less cost effective because of the lower incidence of breast cancer in these women and the high proportion of false positive screening results. In Europe the consensus view is that mammographic screening of younger women on a population basis cannot be justified. In the United Kingdom screening is by invitation from age 50 to 70 inclusive.

Frequency of screening

In the United Kingdom the interval between mammographic screens was selected from evidence from the Swedish two counties study and is every three years. A UKCCCR trial comparing annual with standard triennial mammographic screens has shown a small and insignificant advantage for annual screening of women. Screening needs to be shorter than the mean sojourn time for age. For women over 60 an interval of three years seems to be effective. For women aged 50–60, the ideal screening interval is probably between two and three years. If screening is offered to women aged <50, it should be annual.

Screening method

There is clear evidence that two mammographic views of each breast (mediolateral oblique and craniocaudal) significantly improve both sensitivity, particularly for small breast cancers, and specificity. A comparison of performance in UK screening units showed a 42% increase in the detection of carcinomas measuring <15 mm in units that use two views. Data from the UK screening programme also indicate significant improvements in detection rates of small cancers when the mammographic film density is between 1.5 and 1.9. Double reading of films improves sensitivity by 5–10%.

Expected results from screening 10 000 women

	No of women
First prevalent screening, women aged 50–52	
Women screened	10 000
Recall for assessment	700–1000
Invasive cancers found	27–36
Small invasive cancers found (<15 mm)	15–20
Carcinoma in situ	4
Benign surgical biopsies	18–36
Repeat (incident) screen, women aged 53–70	
Women screened	10 000
Recalled for assessment	500–700
Invasive cancers found	31–42
Small invasive cancers found (<15 mm)	17–23
Carcinoma in situ	5
Benign surgical biopsies	10–20

The screening process

The first part of screening is the basic screen. The radiologist is responsible for ensuring appropriate levels of sensitivity and specificity. Among women aged 50–52, a minimum of 36

Results from the NHSBSP 2001–2 in women aged > 50

	No of women
Total No of women invited (includes early recalls)	1 752 526
Acceptance rate (% of invited)	75.5
No of women screened (invited)	1 323 968
No of women screened (self/GP referrals)	137 549
Total No of women screened	1 461 517
No of women recalled for assessment	77 911
% of women screened recalled for assessment	5.3
No of benign surgical biopsies	1930
Total No of cancers detected	10 003
Total cancers detected per 1000 women screened	6.8
No of in situ cancers detected	2143
No of invasive cancers less than 15 mm	4159
Standardised detection ratio	1.22

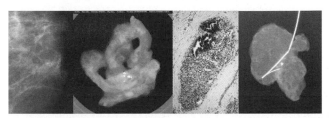

Screening mammogram (left) showing a small cluster of suspicious microcalcifications, (left middle) core biopsy specimen radiograph showing satisfactory sampling, (right middle) histology showing comedo DCIS, and (right) the excised specimen radiograph showing complete excision of this small focus of DCIS

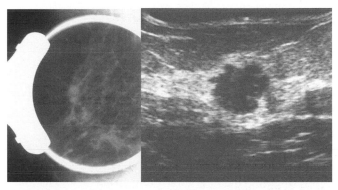

Further assessment mammogram (left) and ultrasound picture showing the typical features of a small carcinoma (right)

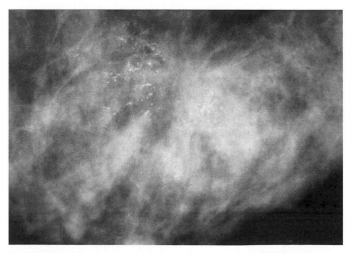

Microcalcifications representing screen detected high grade ductal carcinoma in situ

invasive cancers and four ductal in situ cancers (DCIS) should
be detected for every 10 000 women who attend an initial
(prevalent) screen. At subsequent screens (at ages 53–70) at
least 42 screen detected invasive cancers and five DCIS per
10 000 are expected. More than 55% of all invasive cancers
detected should be less than 15 mm in diameter (measured
pathologically). Recall rates for assessment should be less than
7% among prevalent attendees and less than 5% at subsequent
screens. Women with a "normal" screening outcome should be
informed of their result by letter within two weeks. Patients
judged to have an important abnormality require further
assessment.

There are only two possible end points to assessment: no
relevant abnormality or a diagnosis of breast cancer. Assessment
should be by the triple approach, combining further imaging
(mammography and ultrasonography) with clinical
examination and proceeding to needle biopsy where indicated.
A dedicated team should carry out assessments. The team
should include radiologists, surgeons, and pathologists and be
supported by specialist imaging and breast care nursing.

About two thirds of screen detected abnormalities prove to
be unimportant on further mammography or ultrasonography.
When an important abnormality is thought to be present,
diagnosis by needle biopsy should be attempted after clinical
assessment. Up to 70% of important abnormalities detected by
screening are impalpable, and image guided biopsy is
necessary. Automated wide bore (14 gauge) needle core biopsy
is the preferred method as it provides a histological diagnosis,
which has the advantage of differentiating invasive from in situ
disease and can provide an indication of grade. Where
immediate reporting is required fine needle aspiration may be
preferred, but this method generally has lower sensitivity than
core techniques.

Vacuum assisted mammotomy (VAM) is increasingly being
used to sample suspicious microcalcifications and other
abnormalities where there is likely to be diagnostic uncertainty.
VAM will understage DCIS and invasive disease in about 10%
of cases compared with 20% for core biopsy. VAM can also be
used to excise papillary and mucocele-like lesions and avoid the
need for surgical excision.

Cores of microcalcifications should be x rayed to ensure
enough representative material has been sampled. Image
guided biopsy of impalpable lesion using ultrasonography, or
x ray stereotaxis, for abnormalities not visible on
ultrasonography, is highly accurate. Impalpable lesions may be
localised by ultrasonography if visible on this modality or by
mammography. Ultrasound guided biopsy is the method of
choice as it is more accurate, quicker, easier to perform,
cheaper, and associated with less discomfort for the patient
than x ray guided techniques. Ultrasonography is also an
accurate means of performing needle biopsy of palpable
abnormalities. Most benign lesions can be diagnosed with these
needle techniques, and open surgery to establish a diagnosis
should be avoided. For malignant lesions definitive
preoperative diagnosis can be achieved in over 95% of invasive
cancers. The minimum standard for preoperative diagnosis of
cancers in the NHSBSP is 80%.

Needle sampling of palpable lesions is usually carried out
freehand but can be image guided if there is doubt that the
palpable lesion coincides with the radiological abnormality.
Image guided biopsy should be attempted if the first freehand
biopsy fails to achieve a definitive diagnosis. Diagnostic open
surgical biopsy is indicated when two separate attempts at
needle sampling of suspicious lesions have failed to provide a
definitive diagnosis.

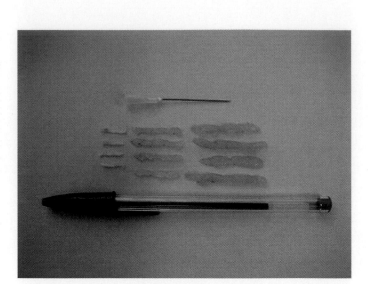
Comparative sizes of 18, 14, and 11 gauge core specimens, yielding on average 17, 100, and 300 mg of tissue per core, respectively

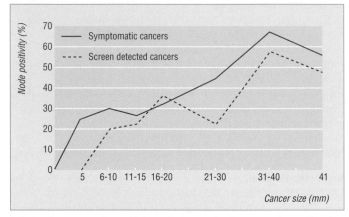
Relation between node positivity and tumour size for screen detected and symptomatic breast cancers

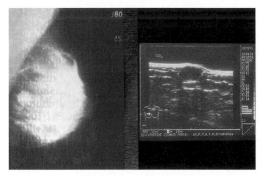
Discrete lesion identified on screening. Ultrasound examination of the lesion showed it to be benign

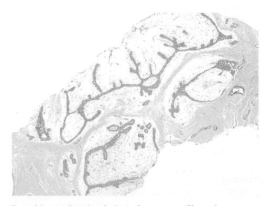
Core biopsy showing lesion above was a fibroadenoma

Multidisciplinary assessment

When results of all diagnostic procedures are available, the multidisciplinary team should discuss these together and decide on appropriate management. Preoperative diagnosis of cancer facilitates informed patient counselling and choice of treatments, it also allows the surgeon to plan definitive treatment as a one stage surgical procedure in most patients and avoids the need for frozen section.

Localisation biopsy and excision

Impalpable lesions need to be localised for surgery. This can be achieved by using image guidance to place a hooked wire in the tissues adjacent to the lesion. The surgeon can then identify the site of the abnormality and excise it. Accurate placement of the localising wire is essential. Various systems are available. Radiolabelled occult lesion localisation (ROLL) is an alternative method to wire marking and may be associated with less discomfort. Superficial lesions can also be effectively localised by skin marking.

If the procedure is being performed to establish a diagnosis, a representative portion of the lesion is excised through a small incision, so leaving a satisfactory cosmetic result if the lesion proves to be benign (the European surgical quality assurance guidelines require such diagnostic surgical excision specimens to weigh < 30 g). In therapeutic excisions the lesion should be excised with a 10 mm macroscopic margin of normal tissue. Intraoperative specimen radiography is essential, to check that the lesion has been removed and, if cancer has been diagnosed, to ensure an adequate wide local excision.

Screening high risk groups

Women who are at high risk of developing breast cancer due to family history, previous radiotherapy (for example, mantle radiotherapy for Hodgkin's lymphoma), or benign lesions (atypical hyperplasia) may be selected for screening at young age. However, no screening test has yet been shown to reduce mortality in such women. Screening should not be offered to those at minimal increased risk (less than three times the relative risk by age 50).

Methods of screening young women at high risk

Mammography has a greater positive predictive value in young women at high risk compared with age matched controls but it lacks sensitivity. This may be a particular problem in women with BRCA1 mutations. Ultrasound screening significantly improves sensitivity when there is a dense mammographic background pattern but has a lower positive predictive value. Magnetic resonance imaging (MRI) seems the most sensitive method of imaging young women but is expensive. It can detect cancers that are missed by mammography and has a role in screening young women carrying a BRCA1 or 2 mutation. Whichever imaging method is selected it should be repeated annually.

Age to start screening in young women at risk

The age for starting screening should be based on risk rather than the age of affected relatives. For women at high risk (more than four times the relative risk by age 50) screening can be started at age 30-35. For those at moderate risk (three to four times the risk by age 50) screening should start at age 40. In each case screening should be annual and women must be advised about the limitations and risks of screening at young age.

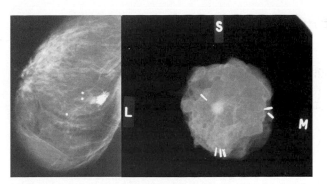

Mammogram showing (left) iodinated contrast marking the site of injections for ROLL using high molecular weight colloid and (right) subsequent radiograph of specimen confirming satisfactory surgical excision

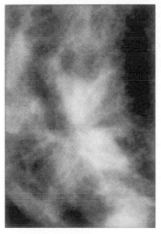

Where small areas of calcification are biopsied, a marker should be inserted. In this ultrasound picture gel pellets were placed at the site of recent stereotaxis core biopsy to allow for localisation for surgery with ultrasonography

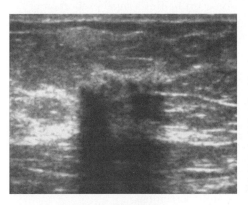
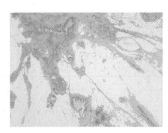

Impalpable stellate lesion detected by screening. Lesion is either a radial scar or an invasive carcinoma and so biopsy is required

Histology of the lesion showed a radial scar (low power view)

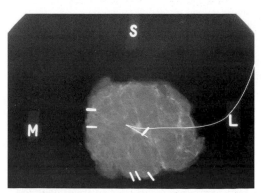

Oriented specimen radiograph of therapeutic excision showing adequate excision at all lateral margins. (S = superior, M = medial, L = lateral)

Benefits and potential drawbacks of screening

Characteristics of screen detected cancers

Compared with symptomatic cancers, those detected by screening are smaller and are more likely to be non-invasive (in situ), while any invasive cancers detected are more likely to be better differentiated, of special type, and node negative. The ability of screening to affect mortality from breast cancer indicates that early diagnosis identifies breast cancers at an earlier stage in their evolution when the chance of metastatic disease being present is smaller. Inevitably mammographic screening will result in overdiagnosis of cancers that may have never developed to a life threatening stage, such as low grade ductal carcinoma in situ. Current evaluation, however, suggests that such overdiagnosis occurs in only a small proportion of cases and that the overall benefits far exceed the potential harm. Women should, however, be fully informed of both the potential benefits and harms associated with mammographic screening.

The effectiveness of mammographic screening is influenced by several factors. A dense background pattern on mammography significantly reduces the sensitivity of screening. The sensitivity of mammography for malignancy is as high as 98% where the background pattern is fatty but this falls to less than 50% in the dense breast. Younger age and use of hormone replacement therapy are independently associated with increased mammographic density and hence reduced sensitivity of mammographic screening.

Breast cancer in a woman with the BRCA1 susceptibility gene is more likely to be occult on mammography as it tends to be high grade and rapidly growing, typically producing little desmoplastic reaction in the surrounding breast and often not associated with microcalcification. Recent evidence suggests that mammography may not be suitable for screening women with the BRCA1 gene and that magnetic resonance imaging is preferable.

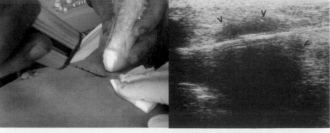

Ultrasound guided biopsy of an impalpable lump in the upper right breast (left) and scan showing needle in lesion (right)

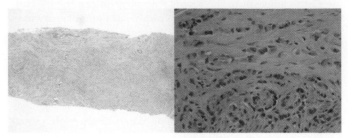

Core biopsy specimen at low (left) and high (right) power, showing invasive lobular carcinoma

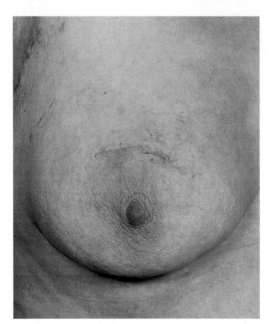

Cosmetic result of recent diagnostic excision biopsy, showing small scar and no visible loss of tissue

---

Histological types of screen detected and symptomatic breast cancers

Type	Screen detected carcinoma
Non-invasive	21%
Invasive:	
Special type*	27%
No special type	52%

*These have a better prognosis than cancers of no special type and include invasive tubular, cribiform, medullary, mucoid, papillary, and microinvasive cancers

Psychological morbidity induced by screening

Invitation to breast screening can lead to some anxiety. There does seem to be a short term increase in anxiety associated with recall for assessment, but three months later, women who are shown to have no important abnormality (false positives) are no more anxious than control women. The excess years as a breast cancer patient caused by a cancer being diagnosed earlier might diminish a patient's quality of life, but the psychological morbidity in women with breast cancer detected by screening has been reported to be similar to or less than that in age matched controls.

Percentage of invasive cancers

	Screen detected (n = 150)	Symptomatic presentation (n = 306)
Grade:		
I	26	12
II	38	35
III	36	54
Lymph node:		
Negative	80	58
Positive	20	41
Median size (mm)	15	20
Nottingham prognostic index:		
Good	46	24
Moderate	48	53
Poor	5	22

Risks of mammography

It has been calculated that for every two million women aged over 50 who have been screened by means of a single mammogram, one extra cancer a year after 10 years may be caused by the radiation delivered to the breast. Compared with an incidence of breast cancer that approaches 2000 in every million women aged 60, this risk is very small.

Unnecessary biopsies

Some women who undergo biopsy will be found not to have cancer, but in Britain the number of women undergoing a biopsy for benign disease is small. The proportion of such biopsies performed in a screening programme should be monitored and compared with that in an unscreened group of women of the same age. Women who require biopsy are likely to be extremely anxious, but there is no evidence that this anxiety is sustained if the results are benign.

The sources of the data presented in illustrations are: JM Dixon, JRC Sainsbury, *Handbook of diseases of the breast*, Edinburgh: Churchill Livingstone, 1993:86, for the graph of results of trials of screening; TJ Anderson et al, *Br J Cancer* 1991;64:108–13, for the graph of node positivity and cancer size for screen detected and symptomatic cancers; and the Association of Breast Surgeons at the British Association of Surgical Oncology audit 2001–2. The data are reproduced with permission of the journals or copyright holders.

Further reading

- Blamey RW, Day N, Young R, Duffy S, Pinder S. The UKCCCR trial of frequency of breast screening. *Breast* 1999;8:215 (abstract).
- Dupont WD. Risk factors for breast cancer in women with proliferative breast disease. *New Engl J Med* 1985;312:146–51.
- Hackshaw AK, Paul EA. Breast self-examination and death from breast cancer: a meta-analysis. *Br J Cancer* 2003;88:1047–53.
- Nystrom L, Andersson I, Bjurstam N, Frisell J, Nordenskjold B, Rutqvist LE. Long-term effects of mammography screening: update overview of the Swedish randomized trials. *Lancet* 2002;359:909–19.
- Tabar L, Yen M-F, Vitak B, Chen H-HT, Smith RA, Duffy SW. Mammography service screening and mortality in breast cancer patients: 20-year follow-up before and after introduction of screening. *Lancet* 2003;361:1405–10.
- Perry N, Broeders M, de Wolf C, Tornberg S. European guidelines for quality assurance in mammographic screening. European Commission 2001 (third edition). ISBN 92–894–1145–7
- Wald NJ, Murphy P, Major PE, Parkes C, Townsend J, Frost C. UKCCCR multicentre randomised control trial of one and two view mammography in breast cancer screening. *BMJ* 1995;311:1189–93.
- Kolb TM, Lichy J, Newhouse JH. Comparison of the performance of screening mammography, physical examination, and breast US and evaluation of the factors that influence them: an analysis of 27,825 patient evaluations. *Radiology* 2002;225:165–75.
- American Cancer Society Guidelines for Breast Cancer Screening: Update 2003. *Can Cancer J Clin* 2003;53:141–69.
- Warner E, Plewes DB, Shumak RS, Catzavelos GC, Di Prospero LS, Yaffe MJ, et al. Comparison of breast MRI, mammography and ultrasound for surveillance of women at high risk for hereditary breast cancer. *J Clin Oncol* 2001;19:3524–31.

or mastectomy. At least 12 randomised clinical trials have compared mastectomy and breast conservation treatment and shown a non-significant 2% (SD 7%) relative reduction in death in favour of breast conserving therapy. Local recurrence rates were similar, with a non-significant 4% (SD 8%) relative reduction in favour of mastectomy. Two large randomised trials comparing mastectomy and breast conserving therapy have shown no significant differences in survival after 20 years of follow up.

Certain clinical and pathological factors may influence selection for breast conservation or mastectomy because of their impact on local recurrence after breast conserving therapy. Complete excision of all invasive and in situ disease is essential. Local recurrence is 3.4 (95% confidence interval 2.6 to 4.6) times more likely if margins are involved. Wider margins (beyond 1 mm) do not reduce local recurrence further but do adversely affect cosmetic outcomes. Neither atypical ductal hyperplasia nor lobular carcinoma at the margins increases local recurrence and re-excision based on their presence at a resection margin is not necessary. The risk of local recurrence falls with increasing age: young patients (<35) are two to three times more likely to develop local recurrence than older patients. Although younger women with breast cancer are more likely to have other risk factors for local recurrence, young age is an independent risk factor. Invasive cancers with an extensive in situ component (EIC) were reported to recur more often, but, providing margins are clear, EIC does not increase recurrence rates. Cancers with evidence of lymphatic or vascular invasion (LVI) have about twice the risk of local recurrence of tumours without LVI. Histological grade I cancers have a 1.5 times lower rate of local recurrence than grade II or III cancers.

Factors associated with increased rates of local recurrence after mastectomy

- Axillary lymph node involvement
- Lymphatic or vascular invasion by cancer
- Grade III carcinoma
- Tumour > 4 cm in diameter (pathological)

There is no consensus of the use of prophylactic antibiotics to reduce rates of wound infection after surgery for breast cancer. One meta-analysis did show a significant reduction in infection rate after a single preoperative dose of antibiotic.

Risk factors for local recurrence of cancer after breast conservation according to in situ component (EIC) in margins

Margins	Boston (Gage et al)		Stanford (Smitt et al)	
	EIC+	EIC−	EIC+	EIC−
Positive	37	7	21	11
Negative	0	3	0	1

Breast conservation surgery

Breast conservation surgery consists of excision of the tumour with a 1 cm macroscopic margin of normal tissue (wide local excision). There are lower levels of psychological morbidity with breast conservation than with mastectomy; it also improves body image, freedom of dress, sexuality, and self esteem. More extensive excisions of a whole quadrant of the breast (quadrantectomy) have worse cosmetic outcomes and do not have significantly lower local recurrence rates than wide excisions. There is no size limit for breast conservation surgery, but adequate excision of lesions over 4 cm usually produces a poor cosmetic result; thus in most breast units conservation surgery tends to be limited to lesions of ≤4 cm. About 10% of

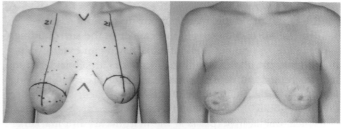

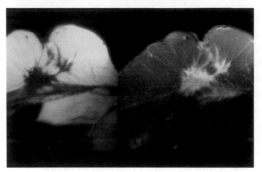

Patient with ptotic breasts and a cancer of the left breast treated with an oncoplastic technique with wide resection of cancer and bilateral breast reduction surgery (reproduced with permission from Miss Eva Weiler-Mithoff, Glasgow)

MRI showing an enhanced and lesion in the breast, characteristic of local recurrence

Risk factors for local recurrence of cancer after breast conservation

Factor	Relative risk
Involved margins	× 3–5
Extensive in situ component*	× 3
Patient's age <35 (v > 50)	× 3
Lymphatic or vascular invasion	× 2
Histological grade II or II (v grade I)	× 1.5

*Not significant if margins are clear

Relation between age and local recurrence of cancer after breast conservation

Age (years)	Recurrence after 5 years
<35	17%
35–50	12%
>50	6%

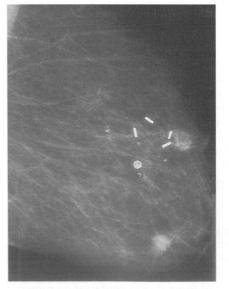

Patient who was treated with breast conservation and developed a new primary cancer in the lower part of treated breast. The metal clips mark the site of the original cancer. About 20% of so called breast recurrences after breast conservation are second primary cancers

the breast volume can be removed without serious cosmetic deficit. There is no age limit for breast conservation. Failure to offer appropriate patients a choice of breast conservation surgery represents a failure of care.

Breast cancers suitable for treatment by breast conservation

- Single clinical and mammographic lesion
- Tumour ≤4 cm in diameter
- No sign of local advancement (T_1, T_2 ≤4 cm), extensive nodal involvement (N_0, N_1), or metastases (M_0)
- Tumour >4 cm in large breast

Factors affecting cosmetic outcome

Around 17% (95% confidence interval 13% to 23%) of women have a poor cosmetic result after wide excision and radiotherapy. Patients with a good cosmetic outcome suffer significantly less anxiety and depression and also have a better body image, sexuality, and self esteem than women with poor cosmetic results. The single most important factor affecting cosmetic outcome is the volume of tissue excised. Large volume excisions (>10% of the breast volume) and removal of skin produces poor cosmetic results. For this reason only dimpled or retracted skin overlying a localised breast cancer should be excised. Where it is evident that wide excision of a tumour will remove over 10% of the breast, consideration should be given to using primary systemic therapy to shrink the tumour, filling the defect by a latissimus dorsi mini-flap, or performing an oncoplastic breast reducing excision combined with reduction to the opposite breast. For patients who get a poor cosmetic result after breast conservation options include replacing the tissue lost with a myocutaneous or a local flap or reduction surgery to the opposite breast.

A central tumour is not a contraindication for breast conserving surgery, and this type of tumour can be excised with primary closure of a local rotational tissue flap from the inferior part of the breast to fill the defect.

Mastectomy

About one third of symptomatic localised breast cancers are unsuitable for treatment by breast conservation but can be treated by mastectomy, and a few patients who are suitable for breast conservation surgery opt for mastectomy. Mastectomy removes breast tissue with some overlying skin, usually including the nipple. The breast is removed from the chest wall muscles (pectoralis major, rectus abdominus, and serratus anterior), which are left intact. Mastectomy should be combined with some form of axillary surgery. The pectoral fascia is not required to be removed.

Patients who are best treated by mastectomy

- Those who prefer treatment by mastectomy
- Those for whom breast conservation treatment would produce an unacceptable cosmetic result (includes some but not all central lesions and carcinomas >4 cm in diameter, although breast conserving surgery is now possible if these lesions are successfully treated by primary systemic therapy or if their breast is reconstructed with a latissimus dorsi mini-flap)
- Those with either clinical or mammographic evidence of more than one focus of cancer in the breast

Complications

Common complications after mastectomy include formation of seroma and, rarely, infection and flap necrosis. Collection of fluid under mastectomy flaps after suction drains have been removed (seroma) occurs in a third to a half of all patients. It is

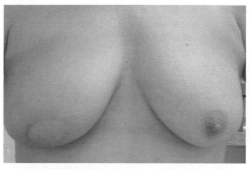

Patient with a central breast cancer treated with central excisions including the nipple and rotation of an island of skin and associated breast tissue (Grisotti flap)

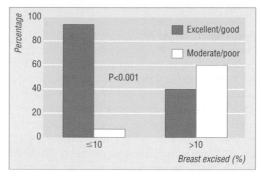

Percentage of good/excellent results in patients according to whether ≤10% or >10% of the breast volume was excised by breast conserving surgery. Data from NSABP BO6 randomised study modified from Fisher B et al. *N Engl J Med* 2002;347:1233–41

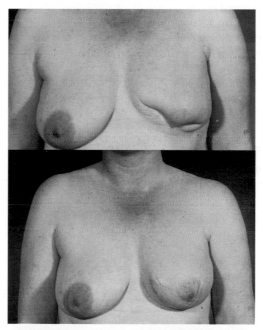

Patient with poor cosmetic result after breast conservation before (above) and after (below) a myocutaneous flap reconstruction

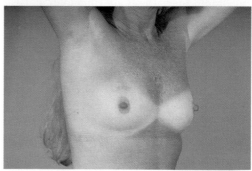

Good cosmetic result after breast conserving surgery and breast radiotherapy

more common after a mastectomy and axillary node clearance than after mastectomy and node sampling. Securing the mastectomy flaps to the chest wall with rows of absorbable sutures seems to reduce the rate of seroma formation. Seromas can be aspirated if they are troublesome. Infection after mastectomy is uncommon, and when it occurs it is usually secondary to flap necrosis or infection entering through the drain site or after seroma aspiration. Treatment is with antibiotics and aspiration and irrigation of the infected cavity with local anaesthetic as for other breast abscesses. Opening up the mastectomy wound and packing the cavity is rarely required and leaves an ugly contracted scar. Most patients treated by mastectomy are suitable for some form of breast reconstruction, which may be performed at the same time as the initial mastectomy.

Follow up of patients after surgery

Local recurrence after mastectomy is most common in the first two years and decreases with time. By contrast, local recurrence after breast conservation occurs at a fixed rate each year. Follow up schedules should take this into account. The aim of follow up is to detect local recurrence, a new cancer in the treated breast, or contralateral disease as early as possible, reducing the need for further treatment and improving long term disease control and survival. Patients with carcinoma of one breast have a higher risk of developing cancer in the other breast, the rate being about 0.6% a year. All patients followed up after breast cancer should, therefore, undergo mammography annually. Mammograms can be difficult to interpret after breast conservation because scarring from surgery can result in the formation of a stellate opacity and localised distortion, which can be difficult to differentiate from cancer recurrence. Magnetic resonance imaging and contrast ultrasonography are useful in this situation. The recent recommendations of discharging of all patients at three years with urgent re-referral if suspicious symptoms develop will be effective only if a regular annual mammographic surveillance programme is provided for all women with breast cancer.

Follow up schedule after surgery for breast cancer

Breast conserving surgery	Mastectomy
• Annual clinical examination for 5–10 years*	• Annual clinical examination for five years
• Annual mammography indefinitely	• Annual mammography indefinitely

*Annual examination to 10 years in women <40 years at diagnosis, otherwise to 5 years

Radiotherapy

All patients should receive radiotherapy to the breast after wide local excision or quadrantectomy. Doses are commonly 40 Gy in 15 fractions over three weeks or 50 Gy in 25 fractions over five weeks. A top up or boost of 10–20 Gy can be given to the tumour bed usually with electrons. Boost reduces local recurrence in all age groups, but the absolute benefit in women aged >60 is small, and so can be omitted in patients aged >60 with clear margins. Newer treatments under investigation include partial breast radiotherapy, either by standard radiotherapy techniques or delivered intraoperatively. A third approach is to put a delivery catheter in place at the time of surgery and to give the radiotherapy with an after loading system in the days after surgery.

After mastectomy, radiotherapy should be considered for patients at high risk of local recurrence which includes patients

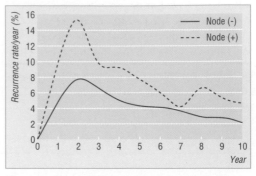

Time to recurrence after primary therapy, Early Breast Cancer Trialists' Collaborative Group. Adapted from *Lancet* 1998;352:930–42

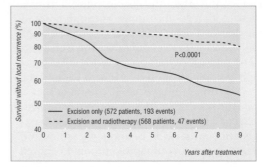

Effect of radiotherapy on local recurrence after wide local excision

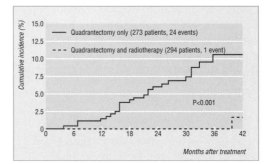

Effect of radiotherapy on local recurrence after quadrantectomy

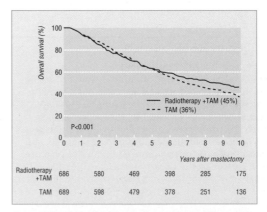

Survival results in the Danish Breast Cancer Cooperative Group trial 82c, comparing tamoxifen (TAM) and radiation therapy (RT) with tamoxifen alone in premenopausal women treated with mastectomy

with involvement of pectoralis major or patients with any two known risk factors associated with an increased risk of recurrence. Although the Early Breast Cancer Trialists' overview showed no survival advantage for radiotherapy to the chest wall after mastectomy, three recent studies that combined radiotherapy and systemic therapy in both premenopausal and postmenopausal high risk women have shown improved survival for patients who received chest wall radiotherapy. The overview presented at San Antonio in 2004 reported a 30.6% local recurrence rate after breast surgery without radiotherapy at 15 years compared with a 10.3% rate with radiotherapy. The biggest difference was in the first five years. Breast cancer mortality was also reduced from 48.1% to 44.0% at 15 years.

Complications

With modern machinery and the delivery of smaller fractions the skin dose of radiotherapy is minimised. This has dramatically reduced the incidence of immediate skin reactions and subsequent skin telangiectasia. With tangential fields, only a part of the left anterior descending artery and a small fraction of lung tissue are now routinely included within radiotherapy fields. Reports of increased cardiac deaths many years after radiotherapy for left sided breast cancer relate to old radiotherapy techniques that delivered higher doses of radiotherapy to a much greater proportion of the heart.

Radiation pneumonitis, which is usually transient, affects less than 2% of patients treated with tangential fields. Rib doses are also smaller, so rib damage is now much less common. Pain in the treated area is rarely mentioned in reviews but is a problem for some patients and may be due to the vasculitis caused by radiotherapy. Cutaneous radionecrosis and osteoradionecrosis are rare with current treatment schedules but are still seen in patients treated many years ago.

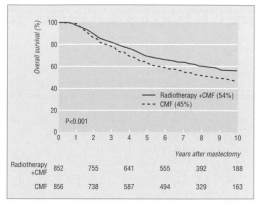

Survival results in the Danish Breast Cancer Cooperative Group trial 82b, comparing CMF (cyclophosphamide, methotrexate, fluorouracil) chemotherapy and radiation therapy with chemotherapy alone in premenopausal women treated with mastectomy

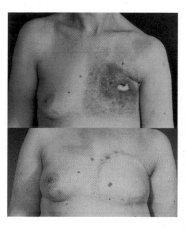

Patient with cutaneous radionecrosis (top) from radiotherapy given over 20 years ago and same patient after excision and pedicled latissimus dorsi myocutaneous flap (bottom)

Effect of radiotherapy after breast conserving surgery at 10 years

	No radiotherapy	Radiotherapy
Recurrence rate	31.9%	10.5%
Mortality	24.7%	20.9%

Data presented by Peto at San Antonio Breast Cancer Conference, 2004. Of 7311 women included in analysis, 6097 were node negative and 1214 were node positive. There was a 3.8% survival benefit (SE 1.1%) in node positive women and a 2.1% survival benefit (SE 1.1%) at 10 years in node negative women

The sources of the data presented in graphs are: B Fisher and C Redmond, *Monogr Natl Cancer Inst* 1992;11:7 13 for recurrence after wide local excision; U Veronesi et al, *N Engl J Med* 1993;328:1587–91 (copyright Massachusetts Medical Society) for recurrence after quadrantectomy; M Overgaard et al, *N Engl J Med* 1997;337:949–55 for survival results in the Danish Breast Cancer Cooperative Group trails. The two graphs of the results of the Danish Breast Cancer Cooperative Group trials are adapted from Overgaard M et al, *Lancet* 1999; 353:1641

Further reading

- Asgiersson KS, McCulley, SJ, Pinder SE, Macmillan RD. Size of invasive breast cancer and risk of local recurrence after breast-conservation therapy. *Eur J Cancer* 2003;39:2462–9.
- Bartelink H, Horiot JC, Poortmans P, Struikmans H, van den Bogaert W, Barillot I, et al. Recurrence rates after treatment of breast cancer with standard radiotherapy with or without additional radiation. *New Engl J Med* 2001;345:1378–87.
- Early Breast Cancer Trialists' Collaborative Group. Effects of radiotherapy and surgery in early breast cancer: an overview of the randomised trials. *New Engl J Med* 1995;333:1444–51.
- Fisher B, Anderson S, Bryant J, Margolese RG, Deutsch M, Fisher ER, et al. Twenty-year follow-up of a randomized trial comparing total mastectomy, lumpectomy, and lumpectomy plus irradiation for the treatment of invasive breast cancer. *N Engl J Med* 2002;347:1233–41.
- Forrest AP, Stewart HJ, Everington D, Prescott RJ, McArdle CS, Harnett AN, et al. On behalf of the Scottish Cancer Trials Group. Randomised controlled trial of conservation therapy for breast cancer: 6-year analysis of the Scottish trial. *Lancet* 1996;348:708–13.
- Gage I, Schnitt SS, Nixon AJ, Silver B, Recht A, Troyan SL, et al. Pathologic margin involvement and the risk of recurrence in patients treated with breast-conserving therapy. *Cancer* 1996;78:1921–7.

- Overgaard M, Jensen M-B, Overgaard J, Hansen PS, Rose C, Andersson M, et al. Randomised controlled trial evaluating postoperative radiotherapy in high-risk postmenopausal breast cancer patients given tamoxifen: report from the Danish breast cancer co-operative group dbcg 82c trial. *Lancet* 1999;353:1641.
- Singletary SE. Surgical margins in patients with early-stage breast cancer treated by breast conserving therapy. *Am J Surg* 2002;184:383–93.
- Schain WS, d'Angelo TM, Dunn ME, Lichter AS, Pierce LJ. Mastectomy versus conservative surgery and radiation therapy: psychological consequences. *Cancer* 1994;73:1221–8.
- Smitt MC, Nowels KW, Zdeblick MJ, Jeffrey S, Carlson RW, Stockdale FE, et al. The importance of the lumpectomy surgical margin status in long term results of breast conservation. *Cancer* 1995;76:259–67.
- Veronesi U, Cascinelli N, Mariani L, Greco M, Saccozzi R, Luini A, et al. Twenty-year follow-up of a randomized study comparing breast-conserving surgery with radical mastectomy for early breast cancer. *N Engl J Med* 2002;347:1227–32.
- Veronesi U, Volterrani F, Luini A, Saccozzi R, Del Vecchio M, Zucali R, et al. Quadrantectomy versus lumpectomy for small size breast cancer. *Eur J Cancer* 1990;26:671.

8 Management of regional nodes in breast cancer

NJ Bundred, A Rodger, JM Dixon

Lymph drainage of breast

Lymph drainage from the breast is via the axillary and internal mammary nodes. To a lesser extent lymph also drains by intercostal routes to nodes adjacent to the vertebrae. The axillary nodes receive about 95% of the total lymph drainage, and this is reflected in the greater frequency of tumour metastases to these nodes.

The axillary nodes, which lie below the axillary vein, can be divided into three groups in relation to the pectoralis minor muscle: level I nodes lie lateral to the muscle; level II (central) nodes lie behind the muscle; and level III (apical) nodes lie between the muscle's medial border, the first rib, and the axillary vein. There are on average 20 nodes in the axilla, with about 13 nodes at level I, five at level II, and two at level III. The drainage from level I nodes passes into level II nodes and on into the apical nodes. An alternative route, by which lymph can get to level III nodes without passing through nodes at level I, is through lymph nodes on the undersurface of the pectoralis major muscle, the interpectoral nodes. The orderly drainage of lymph explains why few patients with cancer have affected lymph nodes at levels II or level III without involvement at level I. These so called skip metastases are seen in less than 5% of patients with affected axillary nodes.

Factors affecting lymph node involvement

Preoperative clinical or radiological assessment of lymph node involvement is inaccurate, with only 70% of involved nodes being clinically detectable. Only histopathological assessment of nodes that are palpable, nodes that can be seen using ultrasonography, or excised nodes provides accurate prognostic information: micrometastatic disease detected only by immunohistochemistry does not have the same implications for prognosis and management.

Lymph nodes are ineffective barriers to the spread of cancer, and metastasis indicates biologically aggressive disease that requires systemic adjuvant treatment. Involvement of axillary nodes occurs in up to half of symptomatic breast cancers and in 10–20% of those detected by screening.

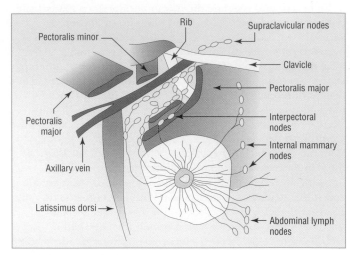

Lymph drainage of the breast

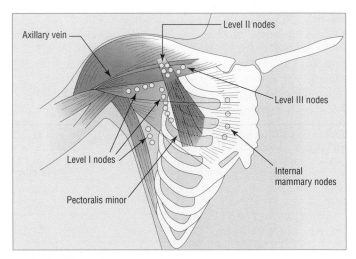

Levels of axillary nodes

Factors associated with lymph node involvement

- Large tumour
- Poorly differentiated tumour (grade III)
- Symptomatic (compared with screen detected) tumour
- Presence of lymphatic or vascular invasion in and around tumour
- Oestrogen receptor negative tumour

Options for axillary surgery

Procedures to stage but not treat the axilla
- Sentinel node biopsy
- Axillary node sampling (removal of at least four lymph nodes)
- Sentinel node biopsy combined with sampling palpable suspicious feeling lymph nodes
- Partial axillary dissection (level I)

Procedures to stage and treat the axilla
- Level II dissection
- Level III dissection

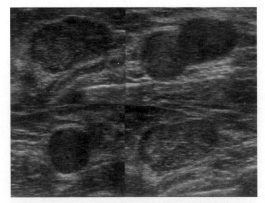

Ultrasound pictures of involved axillary nodes. All patients with invasive breast cancer should have axillary ultrasonogaphy with fine needle aspiration cytology or core biopsy to assess whether any enlarged or abnormal node is involved. Up to half of patients with involved nodes can be detected using ultrasound guided biopsy

Role of axillary surgery in patients with operable breast cancer

Axillary surgery can be used to stage the axilla or to treat axillary disease, or both.

Staging the axilla

The presence or absence of involved axillary lymph nodes is the single best predictor of surviving breast cancer, and important treatment decisions are based on it. Both the number of involved nodes and the level of nodal involvement predict survival. Nodal involvement on routine histopathological examination has prognostic importance, whereas the prognostic importance of micrometastatic disease detected only by examining multiple sections of lymph nodes by immunohistochemistry is much less clear.

A single non-targeted node biopsy does not adequately stage the axilla. Although some centres have found that sampling (surgically dissecting out four separate palpable nodes) provides reliable information on whether axillary nodes are involved, others have found it difficult to identify and dissect out four separate axillary nodes. The probability of a false negative result on sampling decreases as the number of nodes sampled increases. A level I dissection should contain at least 10 nodes to provide an accurate assessment of whether there are axillary nodal metastases but does not provide definitive evidence of the number of involved axillary nodes. Level II or III dissections (removing all nodes at levels I and II or I, II, and III) provide more accurate assessments of the number and level of node involvement.

The first lymph node draining the site of a cancer is known as the "sentinel node." Identification of the sentinel node by peritumoural, intradermal, or subareolar injection of both blue dye (isosulfan blue or patent blue V) and radioisotope colloid followed by histological assessment of blue and/or radioactive nodes assesses axillary node involvement with a sensitivity of at least 91% (95% CI 74% to 96%) and a false negative rate of 4–10%. Subareolar injection seems to have the highest rate of sentinel node detection. In most patients there is not one sentinel node and about 25% of all nodal metastases are not in the bluest or hottest sentinel node. The more sentinel nodes removed the lower the false negative rate.

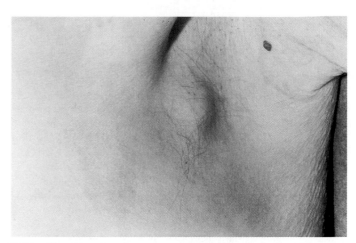

Visible affected lymph node

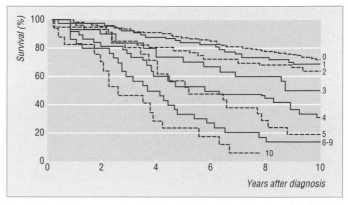

Correlation between number of affected axillary lymph nodes and survival after breast cancer in patients who did not receive systemic therapy

Ten year survival in 368 patients* with T1–3N0 cancers treated from 1976–8 by mastectomy and axillary clearance

Technique	N	10 year disease free survival
IHC negative, H&E negative	285	83% (95% CI 78 to 87), P<0.0001
IHC positive, H&E negative	33	71% (95% CI 60 to 88), P<0.0001
IHC positive, H&E positive	50	50% (95% CI 35 to 71), P<0.0001

*These patients were considered on the basis of standard histological assessment as node negative. An average of 17 nodes were removed. All nodes (2470) were re-examined by standard haematoxylin and eosin (H&E) staining and histochemistry (IHC) at two levels 50 μ apart. There was greater significance if metastases were visible on both IHC and H&E

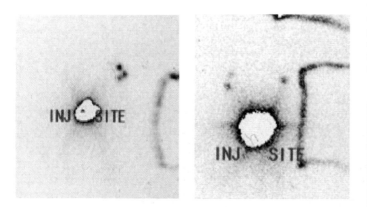

Scintiscans showing drainage of technetium 99m human albumin colloid to show multiple sentinel axillary nodes (left) and both internal mammary and axillary sentinel nodes (right)

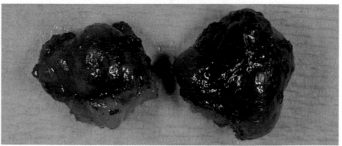

Two blue sentinel axillary nodes identified after injecting patent blue V in the subareolar region

Some surgeons combine sentinel node biopsy with axillary lymph node sampling, removing any palpable suspicious non-sentinel nodes in an attempt to decrease the false negative rate. In up to 6% of patients injected with radioisotope colloid, scintigraphy will visualise a sentinel node in the internal mammary chain. Drainage either to more than one axillary node or a combination of axillary and internal mammary nodes is often seen on scintigraphy. The rate of detection of isolated internal mammary sentinel node metastases is 0.25% or less and is seen with both medial and laterally situated cancers. Debate continues on the value of removing internal mammary nodes identified on preoperative scintigraphy. Removing internal mammary nodes is not without morbidity as an extra incision is necessary in some patients and there is a risk of pleural damage and pneumothorax. Treating affected internal mammary nodes is also a problem as these nodes are difficult to target with radiotherapy. Immediate assessment of frozen sections of sentinel nodes has a false negative rate up to 20%. Intraoperative touch prep cytology misses fewer metastases and has a sensitivity over 90%; it is also quicker than frozen section.

The importance of micrometastases in a sentinel node identified by serial sectioning and immunohistochemistry is not clear. Haematoxylin and eosin (H&E) detected micrometastases <2 mm in sentinel nodes are unlikely to be associated with spread to adjacent non-sentinel lymph nodes. Randomised controlled trials comparing sentinel node biopsy and axillary dissection have shown that sentinel node biopsy produces less morbidity (decreased sensory loss, decreased arm swelling) than a full axillary dissection. Hospital stay is shorter in women undergoing sentinel node biopsy compared with axillary dissection.

Sentinel node biopsy can be performed as an outpatient procedure. Patients with involved nodes are treated by subsequent complete axillary dissection or axillary radiotherapy. Sentinel node biopsy is now routine for clinically N_0 tumours, particularly in patients with small tumours (<2 cm) where the likelihood of axillary lymph involvement is low and routine axillary dissection is difficult to justify.

Treatment of axillary disease

A sentinel node biopsy or an axillary node sampling procedure cannot be considered therapeutic because even if only a single nodal metastasis at level I is detected by standard histology, there is a 12.5% chance of nodes being involved at level II or III. If level I and II dissection has been performed and nodes at level II are involved, there is a 50% chance of level III nodal involvement. Patients having a level I dissection with any involved node and patients having a I and II dissection who have nodes involved at level II require axillary radiotherapy or a complete axillary dissection. Patients with negative nodes after either an adequate sentinel node biopsy or axillary sampling procedure require no further treatment.

Although randomised studies comparing four node sampling with a level III axillary dissection showed a significantly higher rate of axillary relapse with sampling, axillary recurrence after sampling was salvageable by subsequent axillary dissection and survival was not affected. Arm swelling is the major morbidity after clearance, whereas reduction in shoulder mobility is seen after axillary radiotherapy. There is little morbidity after sampling alone.

The morbidity of level II and III dissections is similar and the rates of local recurrence after removing nodes at levels I, II, and III are exceedingly low. Although axillary radiotherapy given after a level II dissection will control metastases at level III, this combination of procedures is associated with high rates of lymphoedema (>30%).

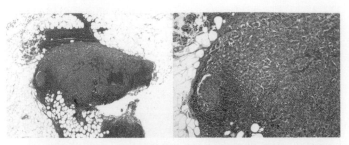

Lymph node with obvious metastases (left: low power; right: high power)

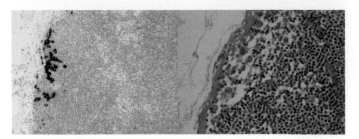

Lymph node seen on H&E (left) and immunohistochemistry (right) for cytokeratin

Current consensus on sentinel node biopsy

- Subareolar injection gives the highest rate of sentinel node detection
- Scintiscans are probably unnecessary
- No proven value in removing internal mammary nodes

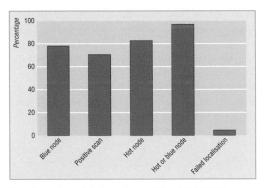

Data from the validation phase of the ALMANAC sentinel node study. Each surgeon completed 40 cases, and data from 840 patients were analysed. This study shows that radioisotope and blue dye are needed to achieve a satisfactory rate of sentinel lymph node detection

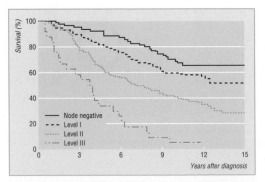

Relation between level of axillary node involvement and survival after breast cancer in patients who did not receive systemic therapy

Symptomatic pneumonitis occurs rarely after radiotherapy to the axilla and is more likely when treatment is combined with breast or chest wall irradiation. The risk should be less than 3% with modern radiotherapy technology.

Control of axillary disease

The options for treating involved axillary nodes are radical radiotherapy or an axillary clearance (removal of nodes at levels I and II if only level I involved or I, II, and III). Both options provide satisfactory rates of disease control, but axillary clearance provides a lower rate of axillary recurrence. Radiotherapy to the axilla cannot be repeated. Ongoing studies are evaluating the need for any axillary therapy in patients with isolated metastases found on sentinel node biopsy.

A watch policy with no axillary surgical staging procedure has been advocated for some patients at low risk of having axillary node involvement, and for patients having breast conserving surgery and radiotherapy because the lower axilla is usually included in the radiotherapy field.

Uncontrolled axillary recurrence, which can manifest as ulceration or brachial neuropathy, is unpleasant and difficult to treat. The aim of treating the axilla is to minimise both local morbidity from the procedure and axillary relapse.

Morbidity of axillary treatments

Damage to nerves in the axilla occurs commonly during axillary dissection but less so with sampling and sentinel node biopsy. The most common nerve damaged is the sensory intercostobrachial nerve; preservation of this nerve during axillary node surgery reduces the number of patients who develop numbness and paraesthesiae down the upper inner aspect of the arm. Radiotherapy may result in brachial plexopathy. This complication may be due in part to overlap of fields, which can result in high doses of radiation being delivered to the brachial plexus. With modern planning techniques, treatment schedules, and newer equipment this complication is rare. Brachial plexopathy can also be due to apical axillary recurrence; this complication is much less common if initial treatment of axillary disease has been optimal.

Wound infection complicates about 5% of axillary surgical procedures and is more common after axillary clearance than sampling or sentinel node biopsy: about one half of patients develop *seromas* after a level III axillary clearance compared with less than 5% of patients who undergo sentinel node biopsy or four node sampling. Closing the axillary space by tacking the skin to the chest wall seems to reduce rate of seroma formation.

Both surgery and radiotherapy are associated with a *reduction in the range of movement* of the shoulder in some patients, and about 5% develop a frozen shoulder. This can be minimised with regular exercise programmes developed and supervised by physiotherapists, and patients with a frozen shoulder require a prolonged course of intensive physiotherapy.

Symptomatic lymphoedema occurs in up to 10% of patients treated by a level II or III axillary dissection or by radical radiotherapy. It is much more common when an extensive axillary dissection (such as a level II dissection) is combined with axillary radiotherapy. Radiotherapy should not be given after a level III axillary dissection. Recurrence in the axilla produces the most extreme lymphoedema. There is no satisfactory treatment for this problem, but symptoms can be improved and, in some patients, the lymphoedema controlled.

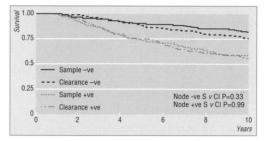

Axillary recurrence rates in patients randomised in the two Edinburgh axillary surgery trials. Patients were treated by mastectomy or breast conserving surgery and were randomised to receive axillary node sampling or clearance. Data from Edinburgh

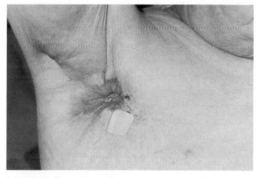

Survival (S) of patients randomised in the two Edinburgh axillary surgery trials. Systemic therapy was given according to node status and not number of involved nodes. Data from Edinburgh

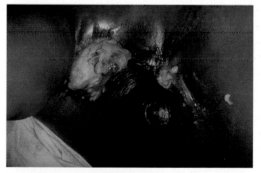

Localised ulcerating axillary recurrence

Ulcerating uncontrolled breast and axillary recurrence

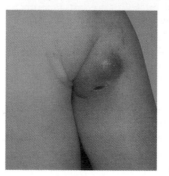

Axillary recurrence causing lymphoma

45

Treatment of internal mammary and supraclavicular nodes

The value of prophylactic irradiation of the internal mammary and supraclavicular nodal areas is unproved. For anatomical and geometric reasons the supraclavicular nodes can readily be included when axillary radiotherapy is given and, providing there is no overlap of fields, adds little in the way of morbidity. Such treatment reduces the rate of supraclavicular recurrence but has no impact on survival.

Over 90% of women with metastases to the internal mammary nodes have axillary node involvement. Of the 5–10% who have internal mammary node involvement in isolation, although most have tumours involving the medial half of the breast, a significant number have lateral tumours. Patients whose tumours drain to the internal mammary nodes can be identified with radioisotope injection and preoperative scintigraphy. There is less drainage to internal mammary nodes with subareolar injection. Internal mammary node biopsy in these patients identifies a small number of patients with isolated internal mammary node metastases but even in this selected group it may still not be worthwhile biopsying these nodes because of the technical problems of irradiating these.

> **Internal mammary nodes can be irradiated only by means of complex fields that include the heart and are no longer routinely covered in radiotherapy fields after mastectomy or wide local excision**

Identifying patients with involved nodes before surgery

Enlarged axillary nodes can be visualised with ultrasonography. Although there are few specific features that indicate that the node is definitely involved, ultrasound guided fine needle aspiration cytology or core biopsy of visibly abnormal or enlarged nodes can identify up to half of patients with involved nodes before surgery, and should now be a routine part of the assessment of women with breast cancer.

Recommended management of axillary nodes

All patients considered fit for axillary surgery who are having a mastectomy or wide excision for invasive breast cancer should normally have a surgical axillary staging procedure. Patients with affected nodes identified by preoperative testing or with nodes considered clinically as being malignant should have a level II or III axillary dissection as this is therapeutic and permits identification of patients with a poor outlook—those with more than 10 affected nodes. Removal of nodes to level II or III during mastectomy allows many patients to avoid further axillary surgery or radiotherapy if the nodes are subsequently found to be involved—this is particularly important for patients undergoing immediate breast reconstruction. Sentinel node biopsy performed with intraoperative assessment or performed as an initial axillary staging procedure is the procedure of chioce for all clinically N_0 patients. Some surgeons combine sentinel node biopsy with an axillary sampling procedure, removing any enlarged palpable nodes as well as any blue or radioactive nodes. This seems to increase the overall accuracy of the procedure while adding little to the morbidity. A second axillary operation in patients with positive nodes on sentinel node biopsy or sampling is technically demanding, particularly

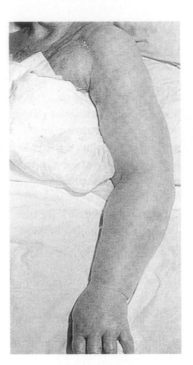

Lymphoma due to recurrent axillary disease

Physical management of lymphoedema

Lymphoedema is chronic swelling that is essentially incurable, though the physical symptoms can be controlled with treatment. There are four cornerstones of treatment:
- *Skin care* is required to maintain good skin condition and reduce the risk of infection
- *Exercise* promotes lymph flow and maintains good limb function
- *Manual lymphatic drainage* is a gentle skin massage that encourages lymph flow and is carried out by a trained therapist
- *Support/compression* with multi-layer lymphoedema bandaging is applied to reduce the size of and improve the condition of the limb to allow fitting of elastic compression garments, which when fitted correctly control swelling and encourage lymph flow

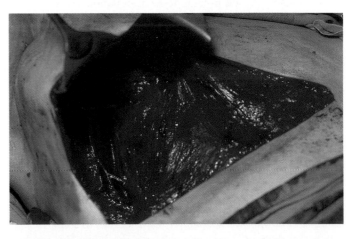

A patient undergoing mastectomy and axillary dissection with preservation of the intercostobrachial nerve

Recommended management of axillary nodes in patients with operable invasive breast cancer

Axillary staging
- Mandatory for all patients

Level II or III dissection
- Patients with palpable clinically involved nodes
- Patients undergoing mastectomy and reconstruction
- Patients with multiple positive nodes on sentinel node biopsy or axillary sampling

Choice of level II or III dissection, axillary sampling, or sentinel node biopsy
- All other patients

when trying to preserve structures such as intercostal nerves and the medial pectoral nerve and vesssels as is associated with greater morbidity than a one stage axillary clearance.

Presentation of breast cancer with enlarged axillary nodes

Fewer than 1 in 300 patients with breast cancers present with nodal metastases and an occult primary cancer. Up to 70% of women shown histologically to have metastatic adenocarcinoma in the axillary nodes will have an occult breast cancer, most of which will be visible on mammography. In patients with no mammographic lesion, MRI will identify occult breast cancer in 70% of patients. Treatment of these women is as for breast cancer with palpable nodal metastases. In the remaining 30%, axillary node clearance (level I, II, and III dissection) should be performed and the breast kept under regular observation or irradiated. Both groups of patients should receive appropriate adjuvant systemic treatment.

Treatment of axillary recurrence

Treatment of axillary recurrence depends on whether it occurs in isolation or in association with other sites of recurrence. If initial axillary therapy has been suboptimal, axillary disease can represent residual untreated disease rather than recurrence. Isolated mobile axillary recurrences should be excised and combined with a level III dissection if this has not already been performed. Patients with isolated inoperable recurrence may be given radiotherapy (if not previously given) or systemic treatment, or both; these are sometimes effective at palliation but rarely produce long lasting control of disease. Radiotherapy given for recurrent disease should be given in a higher dose than is required in the adjuvant setting, increasing acute skin toxicity and the possibility of late side effects such as lymphoedema. Rarely systemic therapy can make locally inoperable axillary disease excisable. When the disease occurs in association with metastases at other sites systemic treatment is indicated. The most effective strategy is to try to prevent recurrence by ensuring adequate initial treatment.

The picture of axillary recurrence causing lymphoedema has been reproduced from NJ Bundred and RE Mansel, eds, *Wolfe coloured atlas of breast disease* (London: Wolfe Medical Publications) 1994 with permission of the publishers. The management of lymphoedema was written by Miss Barbara Lyle, senior physiotherapist and lymphoedema specialist, Edinburgh Breast Unit, Western General Hospital, Edinburgh. The table of ten year survival in cancer patients treated by mastectomy on p. 43 uses data from JM Dixon supplied by Nigel Bundred based on patients treated in Manchester. The bar chart on p. 44 is adapted from data collected by the ALMANAC group, and the two graphs using data from the Edinburgh axillary surgery trials are adapted from JM Dixon (unpublished data) from Edinburgh presented at meetings.

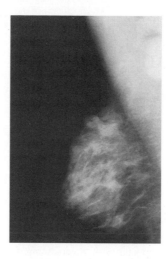

Malignant axillary node visible on mammography with no associated breast lesion

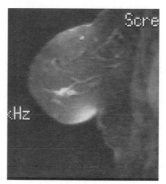

MRI of patient with an affected axillary node but no breast mass. An enhancing mass lesion can be seen, which was an invasive breast cancer

Further reading

- Allweis TM, Badriyyah M, Bar Ad V, Cohen T, Freund HR. Current controversies in sentinel lymph node biopsy for breast cancer. *Breast* 2003;12:163–71.
- Chagpar A, Martin RC 3rd, Chao C, Wong SL, Edwards MJ, Tuttle T, McMasters KM. Validation of subareolar and periareolar injection techniques for breast sentinel lymph node biopsy. *Arch Surg* 2004;139:614–18.
- Chetty U, Jack W, Dillon P, Tyler C, Prescott R. Axillary surgery in patients with breast cancer being treated by breast conservation: a randomised trial of node sampling and axillary clearance. *Breast* 1997;6:226.
- Early Breast Cancer Trialists' Collaborative Group. Effects of radiotherapy and surgery in early breast cancer: an overview of the randomised trials. *N Engl J Med* 1995;333:1444–51.
- Fisher B, Redmond C, Fisher ER, Bauer M, Wolmark N, Wickerham DL, et al. Ten year results of a randomised clinical trial comparing radical mastectomy and total mastectomy with or without radiation. *N Engl J Med* 1985;312:674–81.
- Galimberti V, Zurrida S, Zucali P, Luini A. Can sentinel node biopsy avoid axillary dissection in clinically node-negative breast cancer patients? *Breast* 1998;7:8–10.
- Kuenen-Boumeester V, Menke-Pluymers M, de Kanter AY, Obdeijn IMA, Urich D, Van Der Kwast TH. Ultrasound-guided fine needle aspiration cytology of axillary lymph nodes in breast cancer patients: a preoperative staging procedure. *Eur J Cancer* 2003;39:170–74.
- Morrow M. Axillary dissection: when and how radical? *Semin Surg Oncol* 1996;12:321–7.
- Steele RJC, Forrest APM, Gibson T, Stewart HJ, Chetty U. The efficacy of lower axillary sampling in obtaining lymph node status in breast cancer: a controlled randomised trial. *Br J Surg* 1985;72:368–9.

9 Breast cancer: treatment of elderly patients and uncommon conditions

JM Dixon, JRC Sainsbury, A Rodger

Treatment of elderly patients

About 40% of all breast cancers occur in women aged >70; this percentage will increase over the next decade. Overall breast cancers that develop in older women are biologically less aggressive compared with those seen in younger patients, although survival rates for older women have been poorer mainly because of undertreatment. The average life expectancy of a woman aged 70 is in excess of 14 years and is over eight years for a woman aged 80. Elderly women with breast cancer should be treated in a similar way to younger patients. Few patients are truly unfit for surgery because wide local excision or even mastectomy can, if necessary, be performed under local anaesthesia with sedation. There is no evidence to suggest that elderly patients tolerate radiotherapy less well than younger patients, and when radiotherapy is given it should be given in a radical dose.

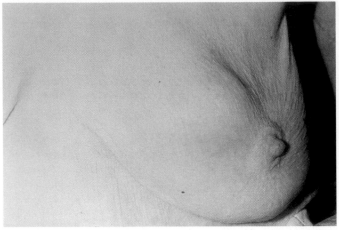

Breast cancer in elderly woman

Management of elderly patients with breast cancer

Tumour stage and size	Treatment options
T_1 or T_2 ≤4 cm, N_{0-1}, M_0	Wide local excision, axillary surgery, and radiotherapy, or mastectomy, node clearance if contraindications to breast conservation or patient choice
T_2 >4 cm or T_3, N_{0-1}, M_0:	
Oestrogen receptor positive	Mastectomy, node clearance, or neoadjuvant letrozole and then, if tumour regresses, wide local excision, axillary surgery, and radiotherapy
Oestrogen receptor negative or no response to letrozole	Mastectomy, node clearance, and adjuvant tamoxifen
T_4, or N_2, M_0:	
Oestrogen receptor positive	Letrozole*
Oestrogen receptor negative or no response to letrozole	Radical radiotherapy or, in selected patients and in those responding to letrozole, mastectomy and radiotherapy; neoadjuvant chemotherapy also an option
Any T, any N, M_1:	
Oestrogen receptor positive	Letrozole and symptomatic treatment
Oestrogen receptor negative	Symptomatic treatment and consider chemotherapy
Very elderly or infirm patients	Letrozole if oestrogen receptor positive. Pallation if oestrogen receptor negative

*Anastrozole and exemestane are alternatives to letrozoles and should be followed by surgery and/or radiotherapy depending on response

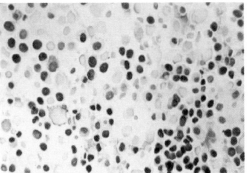

Breast cancer stained for oestrogen receptor: nuclei that stain brown indicate cells that are receptor positive

Operable tumours suitable for breast conservation

Treatments options are breast conservation surgery (wide local excision combined with axillary node surgery, and radiotherapy) or mastectomy and axillary node clearance. Many older women are unhappy about losing a breast and choose breast conservation, and morbidity is much less after this procedure. Simple mastectomy alone is associated with an unacceptable rate of axillary relapse. Although the detection rate of sentinel nodes using blue dye and isotope has been reported to decrease with age, this technique is particularly valuable in older women to limit extensive axillary dissection to

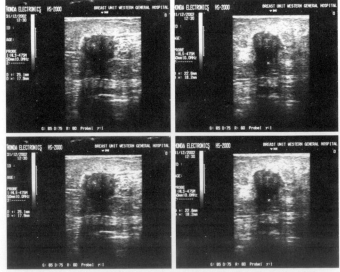

Serial ultrasound scans of breast tumour before and after three months' treatment with letrozole 2.5 mg; tumour is significantly reduced in volume

those women who need it. All elderly patients, regardless of node status, whose tumours express any oestrogen receptor, should be offered adjuvant treatment with an endocrine agent.

Operable tumours suitable for mastectomy

Treatment can be mastectomy combined with sentinel node biopsy or axillary node clearance or, if the tumour is oestrogen receptor rich on core biopsy, neoadjuvant endocrine therapy with an initial three month course of an aromatase inhibitor (letrozole is most commonly used) is an option.

Randomised studies have shown that letrozole is superior to tamoxifen in this setting. During treatment the tumour should be monitored clinically and by imaging: two thirds of appropriately selected women will respond to an aromatase inhibitor with regression of their disease to a lower stage, and over half of patients with oestrogen receptor rich cancers treated with neoadjuvant letrozole become eligible for breast conserving treatment. Response is higher in patients with higher oestrogen receptor levels.

Patients who have not responded after three months' treatment should usually undergo mastectomy and clearance of axillary nodes. Responders whose tumours show evidence of response but remain unsuitable for breast conservation after three months' treatment can continue therapy until the disease becomes operable or suitable for conservation surgery.

Anastrozole has been shown to be superior to tamoxifen in patients who are inoperable or who require mastectomy at the start of treatment. One small randomised study showed a significantly greater conversion rate to breast conservation with exemestane than with tamoxifen. Studies show that local control rates in patients converted to breast conserving surgery are high, providing radiotherapy is given in a standard dose. Without adequate local treatment only 40% of women remain in long term remission on hormone therapy alone.

Older patients have a significantly lower rate of local recurrence after breast conserving surgery than younger patients. Several studies have examined or are examining whether older patients who have complete excision of breast cancer without other relevant risk factors for local recurrence can avoid radiotherapy. Results of these studies indicate that in selected older patients, radiotherapy may not be required after breast conserving surgery. Unless they are part of a trial patients should receive radiotherapy unless there are specific reasons for avoiding it.

Chemotherapy seems less effective in older patients. Several studies have shown that in postmenopausal women with oestrogen receptor rich breast cancers, chemotherapy does not produce a significant survival advantage, although it may improve survival without disease. In high risk patients with oestrogen receptor poor tumours chemotherapy does seem to produce significant benefits.

Locally advanced breast cancer in elderly patients

Patients with oestrogen receptor positive disease should be considered for neoadjuvant treatment with an aromatase inhibitor. In up to a half of patients with oestrogen receptor positive tumours letrozole causes regression of the disease to an extent that some form of local surgery was possible; response rates are highest in oestrogen receptor rich tumours. Oestrogen receptor rich inflammatory cancers also respond to letrozole. Patients with oestrogen receptor positive tumours that show no response by three months should receive locoregional treatment with radiotherapy with or without surgery as appropriate. Fit elderly patients with oestrogen receptor negative tumours can be treated by neoadjuvant chemotherapy or with radiotherapy with or without surgery. Patients who

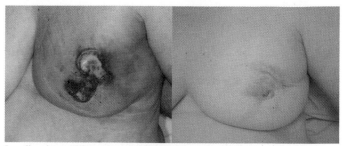

Locally advanced breast cancer showing re-epithelialisation and regression after treatment with letrozole

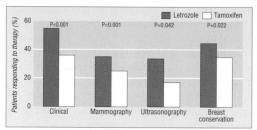

Outcomes in randomised trial (024) of neoadjuvant letrozole *v* tamoxifen. All outcomes were significantly better with letrozole. Adapted from Eiermann W et al. *Ann Oncol* 2001;12:1527-32

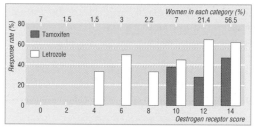

Response in the 024 randomised trial of letrozole *v* tamoxifen related to degree of expression of oestrogen receptor as assessed by Allred score. Adapted from Ellis M et al. *J Clin Oncol* 2001;19:3808-16

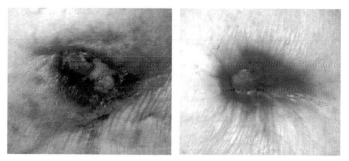

Locally advanced breast cancer showing re-epithelialisation and regression after three months' treatment with endocrine therapy (letrozole 2.5 mg/day)

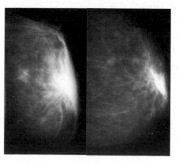

Inflammatory breast cancer showing reduction in breast density and skin oedema after three months' treatment with letrozole

respond to primary chemotherapy may subsequently become suitable for surgical treatment.

Radiotherapy is usually delivered in a radical dose to the breast, chest wall, and axillary nodes with full dose to the skin. Selected patients with locally advanced breast cancer due to direct skin involvement are suitable for an initial mastectomy or wide local excision with radiotherapy. Adjuvant systemic therapy after surgery should be based on the patient's general condition, her wishes, the oestrogen receptor status, the risk of recurrence, and the absolute benefit to the individual.

Metastatic disease

Patients with oestrogen receptor positive tumours should be treated with an aromatase inhibitor. Both letrozole and anastrozole are more effective than tamoxifen in this group of patients, but the data are more impressive for letrozole. Bisphosphonates should be considered in patients with bony disease to reduce fracture rate and improve pain. Patients with oestrogen receptor negative tumours should be treated symptomatically. Palliative chemotherapy may produce a worthwhile response without appreciable toxicity in suitable patients. Palliative radiotherapy to local disease or painful bony metastases should be considered in symptomatic patients.

Very elderly or infirm patients

An extremely small group of very elderly or infirm patients are unfit for treatments other than hormonal agents such as letrozole. These are the only patients for whom these hormonal agents should be considered as sole treatment. In such patients with hormone receptor positive disease if these agents do not control disease, limited surgery under local anaesthesia is possible and can improve symptoms. In patients with oestrogen receptor negative disease, limited surgery to control local disease combined with other supportive treatment should be considered.

Paget's disease of the nipple

Paget's disease is an eczematoid change of the nipple associated with an underlying breast malignancy and is present in 1–2% of patients with breast cancer. In half of these patients there is an underlying mass lesion and 90% of such patients have an invasive carcinoma. In those without a mass lesion, 30% have an invasive carcinoma and the remainder have in situ disease alone.

Paget's disease of the nipple

- Associated with 1–2% of all breast cancers
- Occurs in similar age range as other breast cancers
- Often associated with delay in diagnosis
- Diagnosis established by punch biopsy of nipple

Treatment

- Mass lesion—mastectomy, axillary node surgery, and radiotherapy if indicated; or wide local excision, node surgery, and radiotherapy
- No mass lesion—wide local excision and radiotherapy or mastectomy and sentinel node biopsy or axillary node sampling

---

Paget's disease may be localised or occupy a large area; the lesion should be differentiated from eczema affecting the nipple and from direct infiltration into the nipple by an underlying cancer. Clinically, Paget's disease always affects the nipple from the start, whereas eczema affects the areola region initially and only rarely involves nipple skin. If Paget's disease is suspected on clinical examination, mammography should be performed to determine if there is an underlying lesion. Then a punch or incisional biopsy should be performed under local anaesthesia, removing a portion of abnormal skin, to obtain tissue for

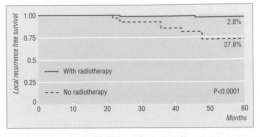

Local recurrence in patients after neoadjuvant endocrine therapy and breast conservation surgery with or without radiotherapy. Adapted from Dixon JM et al. Neoadjuvant treatment. In *Aromatase inhibitors for the treatment of breast cancer.* Ellis MJ, ed. CMP United Business Media, 2005:70

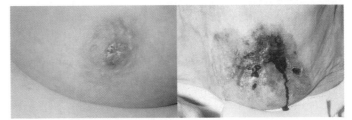

Paget's disease of the nipple: localised (left) and extensive (right)

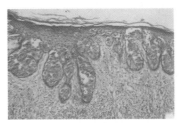

Histology of Paget's disease of the nipple. Clear Paget's cells can be seen within the epidermis

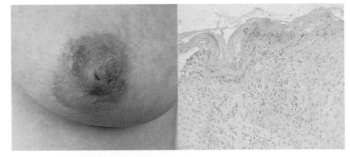

Eczema of the nipple (left) and histology of nipple crusting of the epidermis associated with a chronic dermatitis reaction (right)

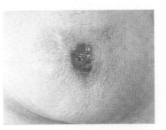

Nipple directly affected by breast cancer

pathological examination. A core biopsy including nipple skin is an alternative.

Management

If a mass lesion is present and is some distance from the nipple, the appropriate treatment is mastectomy and axillary node surgery (sentinel node or clearance—60% of patients with a mass lesion have involved axillary nodes). When Paget's disease is associated with an underlying central mass lesion, wide excision of the nipple, areola, and underlying mass followed by radiotherapy produces a satisfactory cosmetic result and controls local disease. Rotating a local skin and breast tissue flap maintains the breast contour and improves the cosmetic outcome.

For patients without a mass lesion, wide local excision alone if only DCIS is identified followed by postoperative radiotherapy produces satisfactory local control rates. Mastectomy and axillary node sampling or sentinel node biopsy (less than 10% of patients without a clinical mass have nodal metastases) is an alternative treatment and provides long term disease control in over 95% of patients.

Breast cancer and pregnancy

About 1–2% of all breast cancers occur during pregnancy or during lactation, and a quarter of women who develop breast cancer under the age of 35 do so either during or within one year of pregnancy. There is no evidence that breast cancer occurring during pregnancy is more aggressive than other breast cancer, but diagnosis is often delayed because of the difficulty of identifying a discrete mass in an enlarging breast. This means that women tend to present with cancers at a later stage, about 65% having involved axillary nodes.

Management

Treatment during the first two trimesters is a modified radical mastectomy. Radiotherapy should not be delivered during pregnancy. Chemotherapy can be given but is associated with a small risk of fetal damage, particularly in the early stages of pregnancy. Breast cancer in the third trimester can be managed either by immediate surgery or by monitoring the tumour, delivering the baby early at 30–32 weeks, and then instituting treatment after delivery. This allows patients with large or locally advanced breast cancers to have primary systemic treatment, which can cause regression of the disease to a lower stage so disease can be made operable and less extensive surgery can be performed. When monitoring shows the tumour to be increasing in size, treatment (surgery or chemotherapy, depending on which is appropriate) should be instituted before delivery.

Pregnancy after treatment of breast cancer

There is only limited information on the effect of pregnancy on the outcome of a woman with breast cancer, but what data are available show no detrimental effect of pregnancy on survival. It is generally recommended that there should be a delay of two to three years between treatment for breast cancer and pregnancy because most relapses (80%) occur in the first two years. Women treated by breast conserving treatment including radiotherapy have on occasions breast fed from the treated breast with no deleterious effects to mother or baby.

Breast cancer in men

Less than 0.5% of all breast cancers occur in men, and breast cancer comprises 0.7% of all male cancers. The prevalence of BRCA2 mutations in male breast cancer patients has been

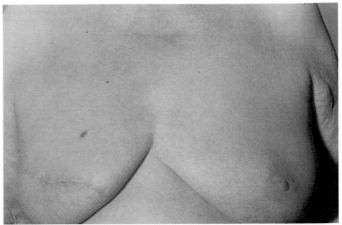

Cosmetic result of treating Paget's disease and underlying mass lesion by wide excision of mass and nipple and areolar complex

---

Breast cancer and pregnancy

- Affects 1–3 of every 10 000 pregnancies
- 25% of all breast cancers in women aged <35 are associated with pregnancy
- 15% of all breast cancers in women aged <40 are associated with pregnancy
- 65% of pregnant women with breast cancer have involved axillary nodes

Treatment

- First and second trimester—mastectomy and axillary node surgery
- Third trimester—either delay treatment and deliver baby at 30–32 weeks or consider primary systemic treatment if tumour is large or locally advanced; mastectomy, node clearance, and radiotherapy if tumour is growing rapidly or wide excision and axillary surgery followed by radiotherapy after delivery

---

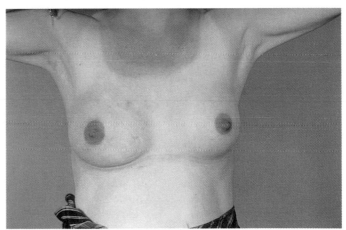

Breast cancer in the right breast during pregnancy

Male breast cancer

- 0.7% of all male cancers
- 0.5% of all breast cancers
- Peak incidence is 5–10 years later than in women
- Klinefelter's syndrome increases risk
- Diagnosis by mammography and core biopsy

Treatment

- Mastectomy, axillary node surgery with or without radiotherapy
- Adjuvant endocrine therapy (usually tamoxifen)
- Consider adjuvant chemotherapy in fit patients if the tumour is oestrogen receptor negative or axillary nodes or both are involved

reported as between 4% and 40%, depending on the population studied, with a mean age at diagnosis of about 60. The peak age incidence of breast cancer in men is five to 10 years later than it is in women. Carriage of a BRCA2 mutation and Klinefelter's syndrome are the only known risk factors for male breast cancer.

Men usually present with a lump or retraction of the skin or nipple. Male breast cancers are usually eccentric masses, whereas gynaecomastia is almost always central. Infiltration of the skin or nipple occurs much earlier in male breast cancer because of the smaller breast volume, and, compared with female breast cancer, the disease is more likely to be advanced at diagnosis. Mammography is valuable in determining whether breast enlargement is due to gynaecomastia or breast cancer. When there is concern that the lesion may be malignant, a core biopsy should be performed to establish a definitive diagnosis. The histology and the prognosis for each tumour stage are similar to those for female breast cancer.

Management

Treatment of localised breast cancer is usually by modified radical mastectomy (mastectomy and clearance of axillary nodes). Mastectomy combined with sentinel node biopsy is an option with or without radiotherapy to the chest wall; radiotherapy is usually given because it is more difficult to get wide excision margins in men and the disease is often locally advanced. Small breast cancers can be treated by wide local excision with sentinel node biopsy or clearance of axillary nodes and postoperative radiotherapy. Adjuvant tamoxifen is effective at reducing recurrence in oestrogen receptor positive breast cancers (more than 80% of male breast cancer is oestrogen receptor positive). There are few data on aromatase inhibitors but they have been used in patients where tamoxifen is contraindicated. Testosterone concentrations should be monitored and a luteinising hormone releasing hormone (LHRH) analogue combined with the aromatase inhibitor if concentrations increase. Adjuvant chemotherapy should be considered for fit patients with tumours that have nodal involvement or are oestrogen receptor negative. Systemic chemotherapy should be considered for fit patients with life threatening metastatic disease or for patients with symptomatic, recurrent, or metastatic disease that does not respond to hormone treatment. The regimens are identical to those used in female breast cancer.

Other rare neoplasms

Lymphomas rarely occur in the breast. Staging investigations, however, are necessary for patients with lymphoma because they usually also have disease outside the breast and regional nodes. Excision, axillary node sampling, radiotherapy, and chemotherapy should be used to treat localised lymphoma. The extent of the excision depends on the size of the lesion. Small lesions can be completely excised, but large lesions should be biopsied as they are sensitive to both radiotherapy and chemotherapy. More generalised lymphoma requires systemic chemotherapy.

Proliferative lesions characterised by spindle cells may range from benign to malignant sarcomas. Lesions in the middle of this range include fibromatosis and nodular fasciitis, which masquerade clinically and mammographically as breast cancers. They are rare but can recur locally after excision. They should be treated by adequate wide local excision and careful surveillance. These lesions are often oestrogen receptor positive and tamoxifen has been used in patients with recurrence. There are few reports of the use of radiotherapy,

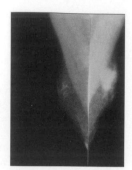

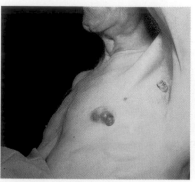

Breast cancer of the left breast in an elderly man. The black mark in the axillary marks the site of the palpable lymph node

Mammogram showing breast cancer in left breast in man

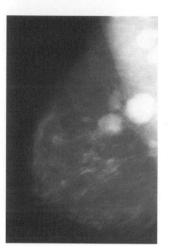

Mammogram showing multiple lymphomatous deposits in breast and regional nodes

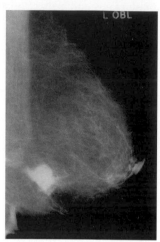

Mammogram showing suspicious abnormality that was subsequently found to be fibromatosis

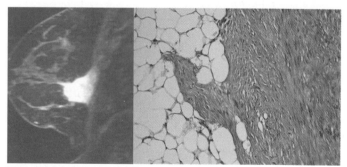

MRI of fibromatosis in young woman (left) and histology of fibromatosis showing spindle cells in a fibrous tissue background and the irregular edges to the lesion (right)

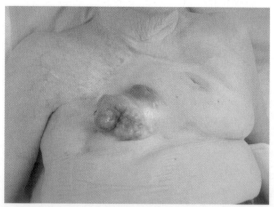

Sarcoma that developed 20 years after radiotherapy to chest wall for breast cancer

but where there is local recurrence that is inoperable, it can delay further regrowth of disease.

Sarcomas may develop in breast tissue or may affect overlying skin, and, rarely, they follow radiotherapy to the chest wall. Diagnosis is often suggested by the results of fine needle aspiration cytology and can usually be established by core biopsy. Sarcomas are best treated by as wide an excision as possible; as many of these tumours are large at diagnosis, mastectomy is generally necessary. Axillary node sampling or sentinel node biopsy is adequate because axillary nodes are rarely involved. Radiotherapy should be given to the chest wall after excisional surgery if not previously used. There is no evidence that adjuvant chemotherapy is of benefit. Survival seems to be related to the size and grade of the tumour.

Phyllodes tumours are rare fibroepithelial neoplasms that range from benign to malignant in their behaviour, though most are benign. Approximately 20% of benign phyllodes recur after excision. In more malignant lesions it is the sarcomatous element that recurs, and almost a quarter of lesions classified as malignant metastasise. Initial treatment is by wide excision, and mastectomy is often required. The role of radiotherapy and chemotherapy in treating these lesions is unclear.

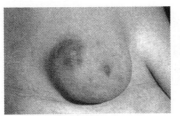

Patient with sarcoma with direct involvement of the overlying skin

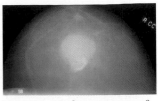

Mammogram of osteosarcoma of breast. Dense bone formation can be seen within the circumscribed lesion.

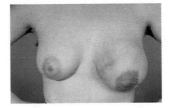

Recurrent malignant phyllodes tumour in left breast of 19 year old woman. Her initial excision had been two months previously

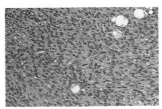

Histology of breast with recurrence of previously excised borderline phyllodes tumour; note cellular pleomorphic spindle celled lesion with frequent mitoses

Further reading

- Anderson ED, Forrest APM, Levack PA, Chetty U, Hawkins RA. Response to endocrine manipulation in large, operable breast cancer. *Br J Cancer* 1989;223–60.
- Dixon JM. Treatment of elderly patients with breast cancer. *BMJ* 1992;304:996–7.
- Dixon JM. Neoadjuvant therapy in postmenopausal women. In: Ingle JN, Dowsett M, eds. *Advances in endocrine therapy of breast cancer*. New York: Summitt Communications, 2004;73–85.
- Dixon JM, Anderson TJ, Miller WR. Neoadjuvant endocrine therapy of breast cancer: a surgical perspective. *Eur J Cancer* 2002;38:2214–21.
- Eiermann W, Paepke S, Appfelstaedt J, et al. Preoperative treatment of postmenopausal breast cancer patients with letrozole: a randomised double-blind multicenter study. *Ann Oncol* 2001;12:1527–32.
- Ellis MJ, Coop A, Singh B, et al. Letrozole is more effective neoadjuvant endocrine therapy than tamoxifen for ErbB1 and/or ErbB2 oestrogen receptor-positive primary breast cancer: evidence from a phase III randomised trial. *J Clin Oncol* 2001;19:3808–16.
- Fargeot P, Bonneterre J, Roche H, Lortholary A, Campone M, Van Praagh I, et al. Disease free survival advantage of weekly epirubicin plus tamoxifen versus tamoxifen alone as adjuvant treatment of operable node positive elderly breast cancer patients: 6 year follow up results of French adjuvant study group 08 trial. *J Clin Oncol* 2004;22:4622–30.
- Hudis H, Tan LK. Rare cancers of the breast. In: Harris JR, Lippman ME, Morrow M, Osborne CK, eds. *Diseases of the breast.* Philadelphia: Lippincott Williams and Wilkins, 2004;1015–34.
- Mustacchi G, Latteier J, Baum M. Tamoxifen alone versus surgery plus tamoxifen for breast cancer of the elderly: meta-analysis of long term results. *Breast Cancer Res Treat* 1998;50:227.
- Ribeiro GG, Swindell R, Harris M, Banerjee SS, Cramer A. A review of the management of the male breast carcinoma based on an analysis of 420 treated cases. *Breast* 1996;5:141–6.
- Petrek JA, Theriault RL. Pregnancy associated breast cancer and subsequent pregnancy in breast cancer survivors. In: Harris JR, Lippman ME, Morrow M, Osborne CK, eds. *Diseases of the breast.* Philadelphia: Lippincott Williams and Wilkins, 2004;1035–46.
- Schott A, Hayes D. Adjuvant chemotherapy for elderly women with hormone receptor-positive breast cancer: an old(er) problem. *J Clin Oncol* 2004;22:4609–9.
- Tretli S, Kvalheim G, Thoresen S, Host H. Survival of breast cancer patients diagnosed during pregnancy or lactation. *Br J Cancer* 1988;58:382.
- Zurrida S, Squicciarni P, Bartoli G, Ravini D, Salvadori B. Treatment for Paget's disease of the breast without an underlying mass lesion: an unresolved problem. *Breast* 1993;2:248–9.

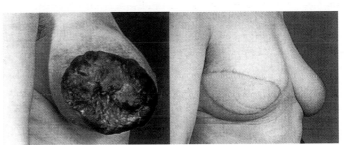

An ulcerated large borderline malignant phyllodes tumour before (left) and after (right) excision and reconstruction

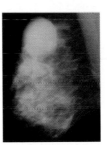

Mammogram showing circumscribed phyllodes tumour

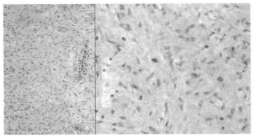

Histology of borderline malignant phyllodes tumour (low power left) and some pleomorphism and mitoses (high power right)

The bar charts on p. 49 from the 024 randomised trials are adapted from Ellis M et al. *J Clin Oncol* 2001;12:1527–32 and Ellis M et al. *J Clin Oncol* 2001;19:3808–16

10 Role of systemic treatment of primary operable breast cancer

IE Smith, S Chua

The past decade has seen an impressive fall of around 15% in the mortality from breast cancer in the United Kingdom, and this has occurred in the face of a rising incidence. This fall coincides with the widespread national uptake of adjuvant systemic therapy and increasing evidence of its benefit for survival. The basis for this treatment comes from the observation that more than half the women with operable breast cancer who receive local regional treatment alone die from metastatic disease. This indicates that micrometastases are present at initial clinical presentation. The major risk factors for the development of metastatic disease are the involvement of axillary nodes, a poor histological grade, large tumour size, and histological evidence of lymphovascular invasion around the tumour site. The absence of oestrogen and progestogen receptors and the overexpression of the HER2 growth factor receptor also carry an adverse prognosis. The only way to improve survival for these women is to give systemic medical treatment, including endocrine therapy, chemotherapy, or targeted therapy with trastuzumab, along with surgery.

Systemic treatment may be given after (adjuvant) or before (neoadjuvant, primary, or preoperative) locoregional treatment. The effectiveness of adjuvant treatment has been shown in randomised clinical trials, whereas the evaluation of neoadjuvant systemic therapy is ongoing. The effectiveness of adjuvant treatment, however, cannot be assessed in individual patients, as there is no overt disease to monitor. In addition, trials that compare different adjuvant therapies take years to produce results; this is an important problem when trying to assess the role of active new drugs in adjuvant therapy. By contrast, the immediate effect of neoadjuvant treatment can be assessed by monitoring the response of the primary tumour to treatment. In addition, regressions in large tumours may allow breast conserving surgery rather than mastectomy.

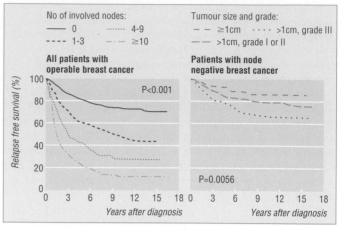

Survival without relapse of patients with operable breast cancer. Data from Guy's Hospital, London

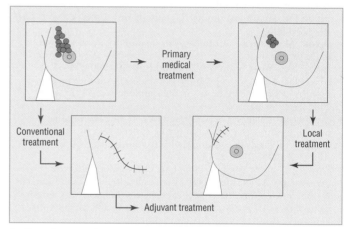

Outline of options for systemic treatment of large, operable breast cancer

Risk categories for those with node negative breast cancer*

Risk category	Risk factor
Minimal risk	Oestrogen receptor or progesterone receptor positive, or both, and all of the below Age ≥ 35 years Pathological tumour size ≤ 2 cm Grade I
Average risk	Oestrogen receptor or progesterone receptor positive, or both, and one of the below Age <35 years Pathological tumour size >2 cm Grade II or III Lymphovascular invasion Oestrogen receptor and progesterone receptor negative HER2 positive cancer

*Modified from St Gallen, 2003

Adjuvant treatment

Polychemotherapy, oophorectomy (including the use of gonadotrophin releasing hormone analogues), tamoxifen, and aromatase inhibitors in postmenopausal women, all reduce the annual rates of tumour recurrence and death. These treatments improve long term survival substantially. Adjuvant endocrine

Data from meta-analysis of trials* that compared ovarian ablation† and no treatment after 15 years' follow up

Treatment	% Reduction (SD) in annual odds of recurrence v controls	% Reduction (SD) in annual odds of overall survival v controls
Ovarian ablation without chemotherapy	25 (7) (n = 1295) (2P = 0.0005)	24 (7) (n = 1295) (2P = 0.0005)
Ovarian ablation with chemotherapy	10 (9) (n = 933) (2P >0.1, not significant)	8 (10) (n = 933) (2P >0.1, not significant)

†All patients were <50 years when randomised and oestrogen and progesterone receptor status was unknown

*Data from Early Breast Cancer Trialists' Collaborative Group
n = number of patient included in analysis

therapies are effective only in patients with oestrogen receptor positive or progesterone receptor positive cancers. The proportional benefit of a specific treatment is usually the same for women at high risk of relapse (including node positive patients) as for women at lower risk, but the absolute reduction in mortality is greater for patients at high risk.

Tamoxifen

- Is a partial oestrogen agonist (has antagonistic actions in breast cancers, but has agonist actions on endometrium, lipids, and bone)
- Is as effective at 20 mg/day as at higher doses
- Is effective in all age groups, and in premenopausal and postmenopausal women
- Is more effective when given for five years rather than two, but there is no evidence that tamoxifen is of additional benefit if taken for more than five years, and it may be detrimental
- Reduces risk of contralateral breast cancer by 40–50%
- May be less effective against HER2 positive tumours
- Is more effective when given after chemotherapy (when this is also indicated) rather than concurrently.

Aromatase inhibitors

- In contrast to tamoxifen, act by inhibiting oestrogen synthesis
- Include the non-steroidal agents anastrozole and letrozole and the steroidal agent exemestane
- Are effective only in postmenopausal women
- Have been shown to improve disease free and metastatic free survival compared with tamoxifen
- Improve disease free survival if patients are switched after two or three years of tamoxifen rather than continuing on tamoxifen
- Reduce the risk of recurrence as extended adjuvant therapy after five years of tamoxifen and improve survival in node positive patients
- Reduce the risk of contralateral breast cancer by a further 40–50% when given instead of, or after, tamoxifen
- Seem to be more effective than tamoxifen against HER2 positive tumours.

Oophorectomy (including gonadotrophin releasing hormone analogues)

- Is of benefit only in premenopausal women
- May be as effective as older cyclophosphamide, methotrexate, and fluorouracil chemotherapy (CMF) schedules but has not been assessed against more effective modern chemotherapy
- May provide further benefit after chemotherapy in premenopausal women who continue to menstruate.

Chemotherapy

Clinical trials have shown that:
- The benefits of chemotherapy are greatest in younger women but are still important up to the age of 70 years
- The absolute benefit increases with increasing adverse prognostic factors, which include number of involved nodes, if the tumour is oestrogen receptor negative, if the tumour has a poor histological grade, lymphovascular invasion, increasing size of tumour, young age (especially <35 years), and if the tumour is HER2 positive, and these factors determine if chemotherapy should be used
- Chemotherapy does not seem to produce substantial benefits in postmenopausal women with grade I or II, oestrogen receptor rich, HER2 negative breast cancer who receive appropriate endocrine treatment
- Anthracycline-containing combinations that use doxorubicin or epirubicin are more effective than traditional CMF chemotherapy combinations. Increasing evidence indicates that the addition of taxanes (and particularly taxotere) to anthracyclines further improves survival in women with node positive disease

Side effects of drugs used for adjuvant treatment

Chemotherapy
- Fatigue and lethargy
- Alopecia (temporary)
- Nausea and vomiting
- Induction of menopause
- Risk of infection
- Oral mucositis
- Diarrhoea
- Weight gain
- Specific side effects of certain drugs

Oophorectomy
- Induction of menopause
- Vaginal dryness
- Hot flushes
- Osteoporosis

Gonadotrophin releasing hormone analogues
- As for oophorectomy
- Pain and bruising at site of injection

Tamoxifen
- Venous thromboembolism
- Hot flushes
- Altered libido
- Gastrointestinal upset
- Vaginal discharge or dryness
- Menstrual disturbance
- Endometrial cancer (investigate any reported vaginal bleeding)
- Weight gain

Aromatase inhibitors
- Hot flushes (less than tamoxifen)
- Joint and muscle pains
- Osteoporosis
- Fatigue
- Vaginal dryness

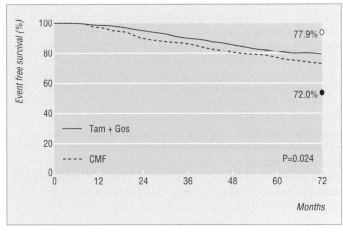

Event free survival at six years from the Austrian Breast Cancer Study Group (ABCSG) V study of premenopausal women randomised to CMF chemotherapy or tamoxifen (Tam) and goserelin (Gos)

Disease free survival at seven years from the ECOG/SWOG INT 0101 study that compared chemotherapy with cyclophosphamide, adriamycin, and fluorouracil (CAF) alone or combined with goserelin or goserelin and tamoxifen

Regimen	Disease free survival (%)	
	<40 years	≥40 years
CAF	49	62
CAF + goserelin	59	66
CAF + goserelin + tamoxifen*	69	74

*At five years, CAF plus goserelin plus tamoxifen resulted in a significantly better disease free survival than CAF alone. No statistically significant difference was seen between CAF plus goserelin plus tamoxifen and CAF plus goserelin

- Accelerated (sometimes called dose dense) chemotherapy given every two weeks with haemopoietic support from granulocyte colony stimulating factor (GCSF) may improve survival further in node positive disease
- Five year survival in women with node positive cancer has risen from around 65% without treatment and around 70% with CMF to >85% with modern anthracycline-taxane combinations.

Side effects: endocrine therapy

The side effects of endocrine treatment are greatest in premenopausal patients. Tamoxifen may cause vaginal dryness or discharge, loss of libido, and hot flushes, and these may have considerable impact upon quality of life (although less than 5% of patients stop treatment because of side effects). First line treatment for vaginal dryness is with a non-hormonal cream (such as Replens), but if this is not effective, locally applied oestrogen should be tried. Aromatase inhibitors also cause vaginal dryness; as even a fixed dose vaginal tablet such as Vagifem can produce systemic oestrogen spillover, caution is required when treating this. Clonidine is rarely effective at relieving flushing and so is not often used. Evening primrose oil has not been shown in controlled trials to produce any significant benefit. Megestrol acetate in a dose of 20 mg twice a day significantly improves flushing in 80% of patients; hot flushes often increase immediately after starting treatment and patients should be informed that treatment for two to four weeks is required to reduce the frequency of hot flushes. Venlafaxine and other serotonin reuptake inhibitors are partially effective for hot flushes but can cause dry mouth. A recent trial has shown that hormone replacement therapy increases the risk of recurrence and so is not recommended. Tibolone is preferable to hormone replacement therapy and is effective at controlling symptoms induced by tamoxifen. An ongoing trial investigating tibolone's long term safety has not yet shown any increase in recurrence of breast cancer.

Weight gain is often reported by women treated with tamoxifen or chemotherapy. Randomised trials have not confirmed more weight gain in patients treated with tamoxifen than those who received placebo. Prolonged use of tamoxifen is associated with a three to four times increased incidence of endometrial cancer and an increased risk of venous thromboembolism in postmenopausal women (although the absolute incidence of these serious side effects remains low). In contrast, tamoxifen decreases the risk of bone loss and osteoporosis, at least in postmenopausal women.

Oophorectomy causes immediate and often severe menopausal symptoms, carries an increased risk of osteoporosis, and is inevitably associated with sterility.

In postmenopausal women, trials have suggested that all the new aromatase inhibitors (anastrozole, letrozole, and exemestane) cause fewer hot flushes, and less vaginal discharge, vaginal bleeding, endometrial cancer, and venous thromboembolism than tamoxifen. These drugs are, however, associated with an increased risk of fractures and osteoporosis. The main short term problems of aromatase inhibitors are joint and muscle pains; these occur in few women, but the pain can be severe and treatment may need to be stopped. The long term risks of these drugs on bone turnover, lipid metabolism, cardiovascular function, and cognitive function have yet to be determined.

Side effects: chemotherapy

Although hair loss is the most common concern of patients before starting chemotherapy, 80% report fatigue and lethargy

---

Improvements in recurrence free and overall survival of women with early breast cancer associated with treatment versus no treatment

Treatment	% Proportional risk reduction (SD) in recurrence	% Proportional risk reduction (SD) in mortality
Five years of tamoxifen alone		
<50 years	47	30
≥ 50 years	45	20
Chemotherapy alone		
<50 years	37	27
≥ 50 years	22	14
Combined chemotherapy and hormonal treatment		
<50 years	40–50	30–40
≥ 50 years	45	30

Reduction in recurrence and mortality in trials of polychemotherapy*

Age (years)	% Reduction (SD) in annual odds of recurrence	% Reduction (SD) in odds of death
<40	37(7)	27 (8)
40–9	34 (5)	27 (5)
50–9	22 (4)	14 (4)
60–9	18 (4)	8 (4)
All	23 (8)	15(2)

*Data from Early Breast Cancer Trialists' Collaborative Group. *Lancet* 1998;352:930–42

Odds reduction of risk recurrence and absolute survival benefits for postmenopausal patients given tamoxifen subdivided by oestrogen receptor*

Duration of tamoxifen	% Reduction (SD) in odds	
	Recurrence	Death
One year		
Oestrogen receptor poor†	6 (8)	6 (8)
Oestrogen receptor unknown	20 (4)	10 (4)
Oestrogen receptor positive	21 (5)	14 (5)
Two years		
Oestrogen receptor poor†	13 (5)	7(5)
Oestrogen receptor unknown	28 (4)	15 (4)
Oestrogen receptor positive	28 (3)	18 (4)
Five years		
Oestrogen receptor poor†	6 (11)	−3 (11)
Oestrogen receptor unknown	37 (8)	21 (9)
Oestrogen receptor positive	50 (4)	28 (5)

*Data from Early Breast Cancer Trialists' Collaborative Group. *Lancet* 1998;351:1451–67

†<10 fmol/mg

Antiemetic regimens during chemotherapy

Standard antiemetic schedules

- Intravenous dexamethasone (4–8 mg) and intravenous granisetron (3 mg) or ondansetron (8 mg) before chemotherapy, and oral dexamethasone 4 mg 2–3 times daily to take home (for three days)

Additional treatment when needed

- Oral granisetron (1 mg/day) or oral ondansetron (4 mg twice daily) for 3–5 days after chemotherapy
- Domperidone 20 mg four times daily (or by suppository)
- Cyclizine 50 mg three times daily (or by infusional pump)
- Lorazepam 1 mg twice daily (useful for anticipatory symptoms)

as the most troublesome side effect. Alopecia caused by some chemotherapy regimens may be reduced by scalp cooling. Nausea and vomiting are unpleasant side effects, but can be controlled in most patients by appropriate antiemetic drugs including the serotonin-3 antagonists granisetron and ondansetron. These should be used as first line treatment, even for moderately emetogenic chemotherapy.

Haematological toxicity (particularly neutropenia) is a common side effect of most chemotherapy regimens, but neutropenic infection occurs in about 10% of patients depending on the regimen. The lower the neutrophil nadir and the longer its duration, the greater the chance of sepsis developing. This requires urgent treatment with appropriate intravenous antibiotics and fluids. Trials have shown that dose reductions or delays in treatment may compromise efficacy, and for this reason haemopoietic support with GCSF should be used in patients in whom neutropenia would otherwise compromise treatment. Chemotherapy induced ovarian suppression with loss of fertility is an important problem for younger women; the risk of this increases rapidly at age >35 years. Gonadotrophin releasing hormone agonists may protect the ovaries against infertility or menopause induced by chemotherapy.

Other side effects include oral mucositis. Some drugs have specific problems (for example, fluid retention with taxotere and neuropathy with either taxotere or taxol), and all chemotherapy requires specialist supervision.

Selection of adjuvant treatment

Choice of treatment depends on risk of relapse, potential benefits of different treatments, oestrogen receptor status, age, and acceptability of treatment to the patient. The risk of relapse relates to known prognostic factors, and these can be used to define risk groups. Age or menopausal status is an important factor that influences the choice of adjuvant treatment.

Endocrine therapy

Until recently tamoxifen was the most commonly used hormonal agent in the adjuvant setting in both premenopausal and postmenopausal women. A major development in adjuvant therapy for early breast cancer in postmenopausal women has been the emergence of the so called third generation aromatase inhibitors (anastrozole, letrozole, and exemestane), with increasing evidence of their superiority to tamoxifen. They act by blocking the synthesis of oestrogen, which is mediated through the aromatase enzyme, in contrast to tamoxifen, which is an oestrogen receptor antagonist. Their efficacy has been established only in postmenopausal women. Anastrozole achieved a small but significant disease free survival benefit (3.3% improvement at six years with a hazard ratio (HR) of 0.83 (95% confidence interval 0.73 to 0.94)) in the hormone receptor positive group compared with tamoxifen or the combination in the large arimidex, tamoxifen, alone or in combination (ATAC) trial. Patients treated with anastrozole also had a small but significant reduction (HR 0.86 (0.74 to 0.99)) in distant disease free survival, but the latest analysis at 68 months showed no overall survival difference. Data from the Breast International Group 1–98 (BIG 1–98) study directly compared letrozole with tamoxifen in 8028 women with a median follow-up period of 25.8 months and showed that patients who received immediate treatment with letrozole rather than tamoxifen had an improved disease free survival (HR 0.81 (0.70 to 0.93), P = 0.003), a better breast cancer relapse rate (absolute benefit 3.4% at five years (P = 0.0002)), and a significant improvement in time to development of metastases (HR 0.73).

Proportional risk reductions after five years' tamoxifen by age group after exclusion of patients with oestrogen receptor poor disease*

Age (years)	% Proportion of oestrogen receptor positive patients	% Proportional reduction (SD) in annual odds	
		Recurrence	Death
<50	92	45 (8)	32 (10)
50–59	93	37 (6)	11 (8)
60–69	95	54 (5)	33 (6)
≥ 70	94	54 (13)	34 (13)
All	94	47(3)	26 (4)

*From Early Cancer Trialists Collaborative Group. *Lancet* 1998;351:1451–67

Risk reduction with polychemotherapy in women aged <50 years subdivided by hormone receptor status

Oestrogen receptor status	%Reduction (SD) in odds	
	Recurrence	Death
Poor	40 (7)	35 (9)
Unknown	30 (6)	23 (6)
Positive	33 (8)	20 (10)

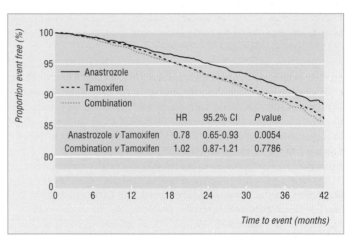

Disease free survival in women with oestrogen receptor positive cancer in the study of adjuvant anastrozole, tamoxifen, or the combination (ATAC). Curves are truncated at 42 months. Adapted from *Lancet* 2002;359:2131–9

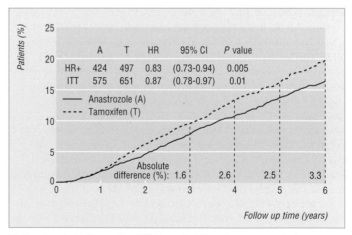

Updated analysis (December 2004): probability of recurrence in hormone receptor positive population (HR+) in the ATAC study. Numbers indicate number of events in hormone receptor population and intention to treat analysis (ITT). Adapted from Howell A, on behalf of ATAC Trialists Group. *Lancet* 2005;365:60–62

These results are similar to those with anastrozole. Letrozole is a more potent inhibitor of oestrogen synthesis than anastrozole, and results from these adjuvant trials are consistent with letrozole having a similar or slightly greater clinical efficacy than anastrozole. A problem identified in the BIG 1–98 study was a small, non-significant increase in the number of non breast cancer deaths from stroke (7 *v* 1) and cardiac death (26 *v* 13) in women who had received letrozole. As tamoxifen reduces cholesterol levels and may reduce death rates from myocardial infarct, any excess of deaths with letrozole could be the result of a reduction in events with tamoxifen. In the ATAC and BIG 1–98 studies there were more fractures, fewer thromboembolic events, fewer endometrial cancers, and fewer other gynaecological problems in women who had received anastrozole or letrozole.

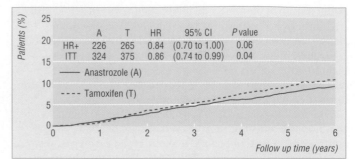

Updated analysis (December 2004). Metastatic disease free survival from ATAC study. HR+ = hormone receptor positive; ITT = intention to treat. Adapted from Howell A et al, presentation at San Antonio Breast Cancer Symposium, 2004

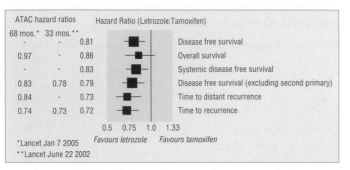

Hazard ratios from BIG 1–98 collaborative study (columns 1 and 2) and data from ATAC studies (column 3) for comparison

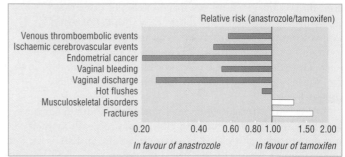

Toxicity profile update of ATAC study. Adapted from Howell A et al, San Antonio Breast Cancer Symposium, 2004

The sequential use of exemestane therapy after two or three years of tamoxifen for the remainder of the five years showed a significant improvement over standard five years, tamoxifen alone, with a reduction in events (HR 0.68 (0.56 to 0.82)), and an absolute disease free survival benefit of 4.7% at three years. A small but non-significant (at the predefined level of significance) excess of myocardial infarcts in the exemestane group again raised concerns about the relative effects of tamoxifen and aromatase inhibitors on the cardiovascular system. Nonetheless, there were fewer deaths in women who switched to exemestane, although this difference in favour of exemestane does not yet reach statistical significance (P = 0.08). Combined results of two trials (ABCSG (Trial 8) and the German Adjuvant Breast Cancer Group's arimidex novaldex (ARNO) trial) have shown that a switch to anastrozole after two years of tamoxifen therapy also improves event free survival (HR 0.60 (0.44 to 0.81)).

The ATAC study suggested greater benefit compared with tamoxifen in women who had prior adjuvant chemotherapy; other studies have not shown this. It also indicated greater benefit for anastrozole in tumours that were oestrogen receptor positive but progesterone receptor negative; results from other studies have not shown a greater advantage for aromatase inhibitors in this group.

The Canadian led MA17 trial showed letrozole further decreased the risk of recurrence compared with placebo when given as extended adjuvant therapy to women who remain in remission after five years of tamoxifen, with a predicted absolute gain of 6% four years after randomisation. Benefit was seen in women with both node positive and node negative tumours. In the final updated analysis, the hazard ratios for disease free, distant disease free, and overall survival in node negative patients are 0.45 (0.27 to 0.75), 0.63 (0.31 to 1.27), and 1.52 (0.76 to 3.06) respectively, and in node positive patients the hazard ratios are 0.61 (0.45 to 0.84), 0.53 (0.36 to 0.78), and 0.61 (0.38–0.98), respectively. The significant survival advantage

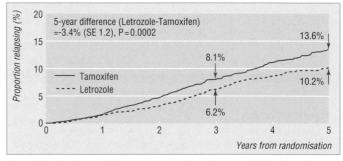

Cumulative incidence of breast cancer relapse from the BIG 1–98 collaborative study coordinated by the International Breast Cancer Study Group. Adapted from Thürlimann B et al, presentation at San Gallen, 2005

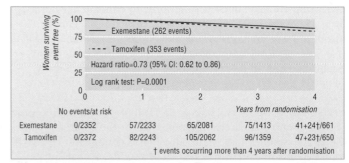

Disease free survival from Intergroup Exemestane Study in which patients were randomised after 2–3 years tamoxifen to continue tamoxifen or to switch to exemestane. Adapted from Coombes R et al, presentation at San Antonio Breast Cancer Symposium, 2004

A recent meta-analysis of all the adjuvant trials with aromatase inhibitors showed a survival advantage for using these agents as part of adjuvant treatment compared to the current standard of 5 years tamoxifen. No excess deaths from non-breast cancer causes were evident with the aromatase inhibitors in node positive patients suggests that letrozole after five years of tamoxifen in oestrogen receptor positive postmenopausal patients will become standard of care for all but very low risk women after five years of tamoxifen. A further randomisation in this trial after 10 years of adjuvant therapy will compare a further five years of letrozole and placebo.

The MA17 trial has reminded doctors that more breast cancer events develop 5–15 years after diagnosis and treatment than within the first five years and has shown that five years of adjuvant hormonal therapy with tamoxifen is unlikely to be optimal. So far, the national surgical adjuvant breast and bowel project 14 (NSABP B14) trial has failed to show any further benefit in extending tamoxifen use after five years and has shown a small detriment with this approach. Two further large trials of extending tamoxifen use beyond five years continue (adjuvant tamoxifen treatment after more (ATTOM) and adjuvant tamoxifen longer against shorter (ATLAS)) and should provide further insight into the optimum duration of this drug.

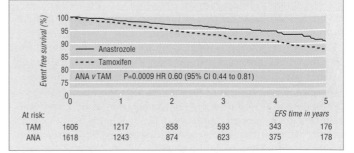

Event free survival from the ABCSG trial 8 and the ARNO 95 study in which patients were randomised to continue tamoxifen or switch to anastrozole after two or three years of tamoxifen. ANA = anastrozole, EFS = event free survival, TAM = tamoxifen. Adapted from Coombes R et al. San Antonio 2004

> **Aromatase inhibitors should be part of the adjuvant treatment regimen of all postmenopausal women with hormone receptor positive breast cancer—ASCO statement 2005**

Adjuvant breast cancer trials with aromatase inhibitors

	No of patients	Follow up (months)	Median age (years)	Node positive (%)	Hormone receptor positive(%)	Chemotherapy given	Hazard ratio	
							Disease free	Survival
ATAC immediately after operation*	6241	68	64	34	84	21	0.83†	0.96
BIG 1–98 immediately after operation‡	8028	26	61	41	99.8	25	0.81†	0.86
IES after 2–3 years of tamoxifen§	4742	37.4	64	50	84.5	32	0.73†	0.83
ABCSG 8 and ARNO after two years of tamoxifen¶	3123	26	63	27	100	0	0.6†	0.76
MA17 after five years of tamoxifen**	5187	30	62	46	100	46	0.58†	1.52 node negative 0.61† node positive

*ATAC compared five years of tamoxifen with five years of anastrozole

†indicates statistically significant difference over tamoxifen or placebo, P<0.05

‡ BIG 1–98 compared immediate letrozole with immediate tamoxifen

§ IES compared after 2–3 years of tamoxifen switching to exemestane or continuing tamoxifen

¶ ABCSG 8/ARNO compared switching anastrozole with continuing tamoxifen after two years of tamoxifen

** MA17 compared five years of letrozole with no therapy after completion of five years of tamoxifen

Ongoing trials

One of the most important of the adjuvant aromatase inhibitor trials is the BIG 1–98, which compares five years of tamoxifen or letrozole alone with sequential therapy of either two years' tamoxifen followed by three years' letrozole or two years' letrozole followed by three years of tamoxifen. A Canadian study will compare the steroidal aromatase inhibitor exemestane with the non-steroidal drug anastrozole.

All of the trials of adjuvant aromatase inhibitor have shown a reduction in the rate of contralateral breast cancers and a reduction in new breast cancers in the treated but conserved breast.

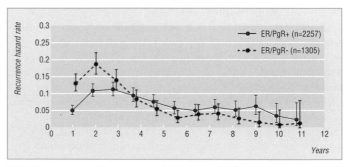

Risk of recurrence of breast cancer in patients who have been categorised as hormone responsive oestrogen receptor or progesterone receptor positive (ER/PgR+), or hormone insensitive oestrogen receptor and progesterone receptor negative (ER/PgR–). Adapted from Saphner T et al. *J Clin Oncol* 1996;14:2738–46

These observations have led to studies of the use of aromatase inhibitors in preventing breast cancer development in high risk postmenopausal women.

In premenopausal women, options include tamoxifen alone or tamoxifen combined with ovarian ablation, most commonly using a gonadotrophin releasing hormone analogue such as goserelin. The addition of tamoxifen to goserelin in younger premenopausal women seems to improve survival in women with oestrogen receptor positive disease. What is not yet clear is whether benefit is gained from adding goserelin to tamoxifen. Trials are underway to compare goserelin and tamoxifen with goserelin and an aromatase inhibitor. Bone loss is a concern with these oestrogen ablating procedures, but it can be prevented by concurrent use of the high potency bisphosphonate zoledronate.

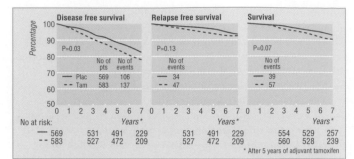
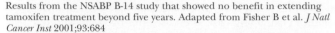
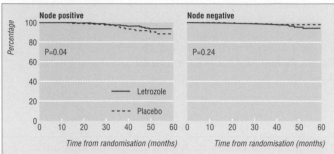

Results from the NSABP B-14 study that showed no benefit in extending tamoxifen treatment beyond five years. Adapted from Fisher B et al. *J Natl Cancer Inst* 2001;93:684

Overall survival in MA17 randomised study of letrozole and placebo after five years of tamoxifen (median follow up 2.5 years). Adapted from Goss P, American Society of Clinical Oncology 2004

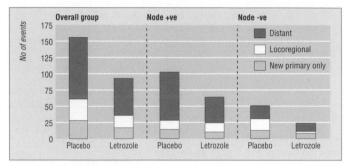

Events in MA17 randomised study of letrozole and placebo after five years of tamoxifen (median follow up 2.5 years). Adapted from Goss P, American Society of Clinical Oncology, 2004

Chemotherapy

The benefits of chemotherapy are greater in younger women. This is not merely through the induction of amenorrhoea (although this may be a factor in some women), as increasing evidence shows that chemotherapy is most effective against oestrogen receptor negative tumours and is more effective in tumours with a higher percentage of proliferating cells; other factors include the dose of drugs prescribed and received. Adjuvant chemotherapy is widely used in women over the age of 50 years, but so far there is no evidence of benefit for those over 70 years. Recent data based on subset analysis of trials in postmenopausal women have also suggested that chemotherapy is of little additional benefit over endocrine therapy alone for oestrogen receptor positive, HER2 negative, grade I or II tumours. Risk benefit considerations are important because of toxicity, and consensus criteria have been defined to aid in patient selection.

Which chemotherapy regimen?

Convincing evidence shows that anthracycline regimens with doxorubicin or epirubicin achieve a significant further survival improvement (around 4–5%) over CMF, and these are increasingly used as standard. In the United Kingdom, a sequential combination of anthracyclines followed by CMF is widely used after it was found to be superior to CMF alone (National Epirubicin Adjuvant Trial (NEAT)), but this regimen uses eight courses of treatment over seven months; shorter duration regimens may be as effective. Indeed, finding the minimum duration for effective treatment is an important challenge in adjuvant chemotherapy.

In node positive patients, two trials have shown a small but statistically significant benefit in disease free survival for sequential paclitaxel after anthracycline chemotherapy, but only one of the two have shown survival benefit so far. More convincingly, the other taxane, docetaxel, given in combination with anthracyclines rather than sequentially, has shown a

Adjuvant trials using taxane in node positive women

Group	Trial design	Number	Survival at five years	
			Disease free	Overall
CALGB 9344	Doxorubicin and cyclophosphamide × 4 + paclitaxel × 4 v Doxorubicin and cyclophosphamide × 4	3121	70 v 65 P = 0.001	80 v 77 P = 0.006
NSABP B28	Doxorubicin and cyclophosphamide × 4 + paclitaxel × 4 v Doxorubicin and cyclophosphamide × 4	3060	76 v 72 P = 0.008	85 v 85 P = 0.98
BCIRG 001	Docetaxel, doxorubicin, and cyclophosphamide × 6 v fluorouracil, doxorubicin, and cyclophosphamide, × 6	1491	75 v 68 P = 0.001	87 v 81 P = 0.008

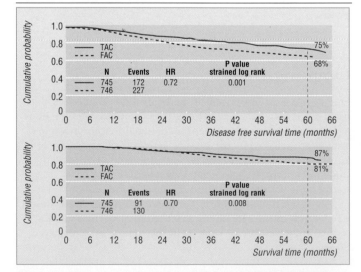

Disease free (top chart) and overall survival (bottom) in a randomised study of adjuvant docetaxel, adriamycin, and cyclophosphamide v fluorouracil, adriamycin and cyclophosphamide. Adapted from Migil M, *N Engl J Med* 2005;352:2302–13

further 6% five year survival advantage over anthracyclines alone. Results of other adjuvant taxotere trials including the British taxotere as adjuvant chemotherapy (TACT) trial, the largest in the world, are awaited. Currently no evidence shows a benefit of taxane in women with node negative cancer.

Recently, a trial (Cancer and Leukemia Group B 9741 (CALGB 9741)) of accelerated (sometimes called dose dense) chemotherapy, in which treatment was given at two week rather than three week intervals, with support from GCSF to overcome the risk of neutropenic sepsis, has shown that accelerated two weekly doxorubicin and cyclophosphamide × 4 followed by Taxol × 4 improved disease free survival and overall survival over the same eight courses given conventionally at three week intervals in women with node positive breast cancer, with four year disease free survival of 82% and 75% respectively. In addition, the accelerated arm was associated with less neutropenic sepsis. The shortened duration of adjuvant treatment associated with accelerated chemotherapy will probably be attractive to patients, and the reduced risk of neutropenic sepsis may save resources. Further trials in this area are indicated.

Combinations of chemotherapy and hormonal therapy

Current data suggest that the use of chemotherapy and tamoxifen together is more effective than either alone for women with higher risk oestrogen receptor positive cancer. Results also suggest that efficacy is greater when tamoxifen is given after chemotherapy rather than concurrently. No data exist on whether the same is true for ovarian ablation or aromatase inhibitors, but it would seem prudent to assume so.

A recent retrospective analysis suggested that premenopausal women (<40 years) who undergo amenorrhoea induced by chemotherapy have a better outlook than those who continue to menstruate. This raises the possibility that ovarian suppression may be beneficial after chemotherapy if menses persist, but this must be balanced against the side effects of the menopause. A randomised trial is investigating this.

High dose chemotherapy with haemopoietic stem cell rescue

Trials show high morbidity and no significant benefit from this approach. This is in contrast to progress with new drugs and accelerated techniques using haemopoietic support with GCSF.

Trastuzumab

Around 20% of breast cancers overexpress the transmembrane growth factor receptor HER2, and this is associated with an adverse prognosis. Trastuzumab is a humanised monoclonal antibody directed against the external domain of the receptor, with clinical activity as a single agent in patients whose cancers overexpress HER2. More importantly, trastuzumab has been shown to improve survival when given in combination with paclitaxel and docetaxel in patients with metastatic disease and achieves high rates of tumour regression with other agents including vinorelbine. Major trials have explored its role as adjuvant therapy in HER2 positive early breast cancer, and these have shown an improvement in disease free survival. Trastuzumab will soon become a common component of adjuvant therapy programmes for most women whose tumours overexpress erb-B2 or HER2.

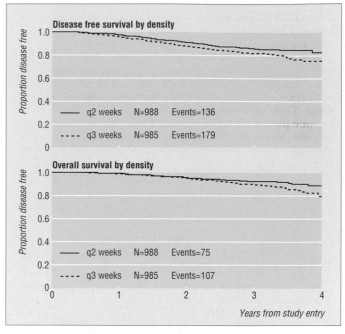

Data from CALGB 9741 study of dose density: (top) disease free survival by dose density; (bottom) overall survival by dose density. Adapted from Citron M et al. *J Clin Oncol* 2003;21:1431–9

Protocol for use of adjuvant aromatase inhibitors in postmenopausal women with operable hormone receptor positive breast cancer

Consider immediate anastrozole/letrozole for
- More than three positive nodes
- Grade III and 1–3 nodes positive
- Oestrogen receptor poor
- HER2 positive

Consider a switch to exemestane or anastrozole after two years of tamoxifen
- All remaining women except those with grade I node negative cancer

Consider letrozole after five years of tamoxifen
- All women who complete five years of tamoxifen except those with grade I node negative cancer

---

Use of adjuvant chemotherapy for patients with operable breast cancer

These factors positively influence the use of chemotherapy:
- Axillary node positivity
- Tumour size (>2 cm)

Histological features:
- Grade III
- Lympho or vascular invasion
- Oestrogen receptor negative and progesterone receptor negative tumours
- Young age (<35 years)
- Strong HER2 overexpression

> In the HERA study, 5100 HER2 positive patients were enrolled at 480 sites in 39 countries. This study randomised patients to standard adjuvant systemic treatment with or without trastuzumab every three weeks for 12–24 months. Follow up results at one year showed a significant 46% reduction in the risk of recurrence of cancer and a 33% reduction in the risk of death. These data indicate that trastuzumab should become part of the adjuvant systemic therapy regimen of patients with HER2 positive breast cancer
> *Presented at American Society of Clinical Oncology, June 2005*

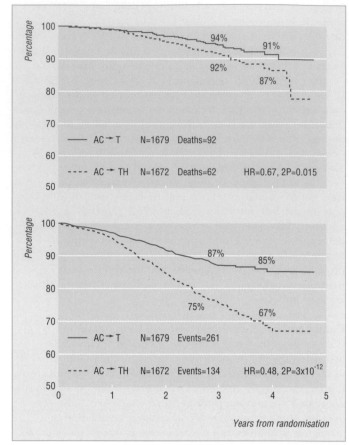

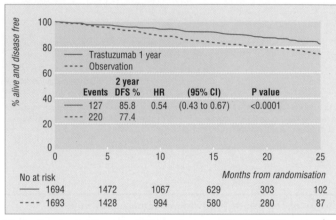

Disease free survival from the HERA study that randomised 5100 women to standard adjuvant therapy (with or without three weekly trastuzumab for one or two years. Data shown relate to patients that received one year of treatment. (DFS = disease free survival). Presented at American Society of Clinical Oncology, 2005

Overall (top chart) and disease free survival (bottom) from NSABP B31 and NCCTG 9831 trials that compared adjuvant chemotherapy in women with cancers positive for HER2. (AC = adriamycin and cyclophosphamide, T = docetaxel, TH = paclitaxel + trastuzumab). Presented at American Society of Clinical Oncology, 2005

Bisphosphonates

Bisphosphonates are drugs that inhibit bone resorption induced by tumours. Recent adjuvant trials indicate that two years of oral clodronate reduces the incidence of bone metastases. One trial shows a small, but significant, improvement in overall survival. Further adjuvant trials are underway with clodronate and the newer, more potent bisphosphonate zoledronate to define their long term effectiveness. Bisphosphonates seem to reduce the bone loss associated with use of aromatase inhibitors. Patients who receive an immediate aromatase inhibitor should have a baseline dual energy x ray absorptiometry scan to check bone density and a follow-up scan after two years. They should also be considered for bisphosphonate therapy if there is significant osteoporosis at diagnosis or major bone loss during treatment. Patients who switch to an aromatase inhibitor after 2–3 years of tamoxifen do not have the same bone loss and so probably do not need a dual energy x ray absorptiometry scan.

Neoadjuvant medical treatment

The main clinical aim of neoadjuvant (also called primary or postoperative) treatment for operable breast cancer before surgery is to downstage large cancers to reduce the need for mastectomy. Another research aim is to use the primary tumour as an in vivo measure of responsiveness to treatment. Adjuvant therapy trials are expensive and take years to complete. The research aim of neoadjuvant therapy is to find short term surrogate markers (clinical, pathological, or biological) in small

St Gallen consensus recommendations of adjuvant treatment for patients with operable breast cancer*

Risk group	Endocrine sensitive		Endocrine nonresponsive
	Premenopausal	Postmenopausal	Premenopausal or posmenopausal
Node negative (minimal risk)	Tamoxifen or none	Tamoxifen/ aromatase inhibitor† or none	N/A
Node negative (average risk)	Ovarian ablation and tamoxifen with or without chemotherapy *or* chemotherapy followed by tamoxifen with or without ovarian ablation *or* ovarian ablation *or* tamoxifen	Tamoxifen/ aromatase inhibitor† *or* chemotherapy then tamoxifen/ aromatase inhibitor†	Chemotherapy
Node positive	Chemotherapy then tamoxifen with or without ovarian ablation *or* tamoxifen and ovarian ablation with or without chemotherapy	Chemotherapy then tamoxifen/ aromatase inhibitor† *or* tamoxifen/ aromatase inhibitor†	Chemotherapy

*The use of aromatase inhibitors rather than tamoxifen in postmenopausal women with oestrogen receptor positive disease will increase
†For appropriate selection, see table on previous page for policy on using aromatase inhibitors

trials that can predict long term outcome accurately. In the immediate preoperative arimidex compared with tamoxifen (IMPACT) trial, biological changes in tumour proliferation as measured by the Ki67 levels after two weeks of treatment were shown to predict correctly the superiority of anastrozole over tamoxifen or the combination in the adjuvant ATAC trial. This approach can also identify the optimal medical treatment for individual patients. In the past few years, important advances have been made in neoadjuvant therapy, particularly endocrine therapy.

Neoadjuvant endocrine treatment

A randomised trial in postmenopausal women with large oestrogen receptor positive cancers that would otherwise require mastectomy showed that letrozole for four months is superior to tamoxifen in terms of clinical response (55% v 36%) and breast conserving surgery (45% v 35%). More recently, a similar trial (IMPACT) compared three months of neoadjuvant anastrozole alone, tamoxifen alone or the two in combination (neoadjuvant ATAC) and showed no significant difference in response rate (37% v 36% v 39%). In the subpopulation with large cancers that require mastectomy, however, anastrozole, like letrozole, was significantly more effective than tamoxifen or the combination in achieving breast conserving surgery (46% v 22% v 26%). A second study, the preoperative arimidex compared with tamoxifen (PROACT) trial, which compared three months of anastrozole and tamoxifen, has again shown similar response rates with the two drugs but a higher rate of breast conserving surgery with anastrozole. When the results of PROACT and IMPACT were combined, a significantly greater response rate was seen in tumours that were locally advanced or required a mastectomy at presentation.

A small study of 73 patients with exemestane also showed a greater rate of conversion to breast conserving surgery with exemestane than with tamoxifen. A striking finding in the letrozole trial was that letrozole achieved a much higher response rate than tamoxifen in the small subgroup of patients whose tumours overexpressed HER1 or HER2 (88% v 21%). The IMPACT trial showed a similar trend for anastrozole over tamoxifen or the combination against HER2 positive tumours (58% v 22% v 31%). Taken together, data from these trials provide compelling evidence that aromatase inhibitors (particularly letrozole) are more effective than tamoxifen in downstaging large oestrogen receptor positive cancers in postmenopausal women to avoid mastectomy. They also argue strongly that aromatase inhibitors are specifically more effective in the small subgroup of patients whose tumours also strongly over express HER2.

The rate of complete excision after neoadjuvant endocrine therapy may be greater than that achieved after neoadjuvant chemotherapy. In a small randomised study of neoadjuvant aromatase inhibitors compared with chemotherapy there was no difference in response rates, but there was a non-significant difference in favour of the aromatase inhibitors on the rate of conversion to breast conserving surgery (P = 0.054).

Neoadjuvant chemotherapy

Neoadjuvant chemotherapy achieves clinical regression of tumours in around 70–80% of patients, which suggests that early cancers may be more chemosensitive than metastatic disease. Around 15–20% of patients achieve a complete pathological response of their tumour; this is much more common in oestrogen receptor negative than oestrogen receptor positive tumours, and complete response is a powerful predictor for good long term outcome. Randomised trials have shown that survival is similar whether chemotherapy is given before or after

Results from randomised trial of 2411 women with operable breast cancer enrolled in NSABP B27 protocol at median follow up of 68.8 months

Treatment	Group I	Group II	Group III
	Adriamycin and cyclophosphamide × 4 then surgery	Adriamycin and cyclophosphamide × 4 then docetaxel × 4 then surgery	Adriamycin and cyclophosphamide × 4 then surgery then docetaxel × 4
Complete pathology response	150	143	163
Deaths from any case	9	18	18
Relapse free events	247	210(P = 0.03)	230
Local recurrence	67	43	44(P = 0.0014)

In contrast with neoadjuvant chemotherapy, pathological complete remissions are rare with endocrine therapy, but easy administration and lack of side effects make it an attractive first line option for older women with large operable or locally advanced breast cancers

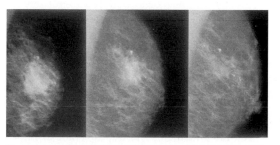

Serial mammograms during primary treatment with neoadjuvant chemotherapy. Mass lesion disappeared, but microcalcification remained; subsequent mastectomy showed that the microcalcification was associated with residual carcinoma in situ

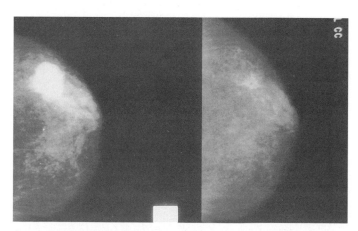

Carcinoma of breast before and after neoadjuvant chemotherapy

surgery. The neoadjuvant approach, however, reduces the need for mastectomy and provides potentially valuable data on clinical and biological responsiveness to treatment. The regimens used for neoadjuvant chemotherapy are generally the same as those used for adjuvant treatment. Continuous infusional chemotherapy regimens are no more effective than conventional schedules, but the NSABP B27 trial showed that four courses of sequential taxotere after four courses of anthracyclines (eight cycles) achieve higher clinical and pathological complete remissions than four cycles of anthracycline chemotherapy alone. Surprisingly, recent results from this trial have shown that this gain in rates of pathological complete remissions did not translate into an anticipated improvement in survival for sequential taxotere usage. This refutes the hypothesis that differences in the rates of pathological complete remissions with neoadjuvant chemotherapy are a useful short term surrogate predictor for long term outcome.

Rates of survival after breast conserving surgery are improved by neoadjuvant chemotherapy, but the extent of the disease after treatment can be difficult to map. MRI provides the best imaging assessment of response. Multiple isolated islands of tumour cells and involved margins are visible on MRI and reported in about 25% of all patients. This contrasts with neoadjuvant hormone therapy, which seems to shrink cancers concentrically, with low rates of incomplete excision and local recurrence after radiotherapy (<3% at five years).

Neoadjuvant trastuzumab
Trastuzumab achieved high response rates in combination with neoadjuvant chemotherapy in breast cancers that overexpressed HER2. It improved pathological complete remission rate significantly in one small trial. It will probably soon become standard care in the neoadjuvant treatment of large and locally advanced HER2 positive breast cancer.

Outcome
Progressive disease during neoadjuvant chemotherapy is rare (<5% of patients); should this occur, there should be a switch to second line chemotherapy or to surgery. Around 50% of patients with large cancers will have enough tumour regression to avoid mastectomy, but all patients still require some form of surgery after neadjuvant treatment, and usually also need radiotherapy (according to standard guidelines).

Selection of patients
Neoadjuvant systemic treatment was initially given to patients with locally advanced (inoperable) breast cancers. Its use has now been extended to patients with large operable breast cancers to try to avoid mastectomy. In these patients, neoadjuvant treatment has been shown to be as effective as standard adjuvant treatment. In other groups of patients, neoadjuvant treatment should be used only during clinical trials that investigate the use of surrogate clinical and biological markers for treatment outcome.

Multidisciplinary teams
The roles of adjuvant and neoadjuvant medical treatments in improving survival in early breast cancer emphasise the importance of patients being assessed and managed by multidisciplinary teams.

The tables on p. 54 and p. 62 using information from St Gallen are adapted from Goldhirsch A et al. *J Clin Oncol* 2003;21:3357–65. The table on p. 55 of disease free survival from the ECOG/SWOG INT 0101 study is adapted from Davidson et al. 2002. The graph showing event free survival at six years from the ABCSG V study is adapted from Jakesa et al. *J Clin Oncol* 2002;20:4621

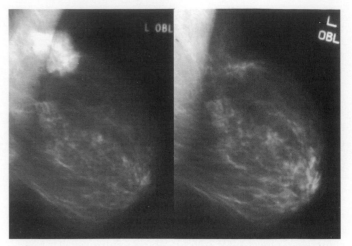

Carcinoma of right breast before (left) and after (right) three months of neoadjuvant letrozole

Further reading
- ATAC Trialists Group. Anastrozole alone or in combination with tamoxifen versus tamoxifen alone for adjuvant treatment of postmenopausal women with early breast cancer: first results of the ATAC randomised trial. *Lancet* 2002;359:2131–9.
- Citron ML, Berry DA, Cirrincione C, Hudis C, Winder EP, Gradisher WS, et al. Randomized trial of dose-dense versus conventionally scheduled and sequential versus concurrent combination chemotherapy as postoperative adjuvant treatment of node-positive primary breast cancer: first report of Intergroup Trial C9741/Cancer and Leukaemia Group B Trial 9741. *J Clin Oncol* 2003;21:1431–9.
- Coombes RC, Hall E, Gibson LJ, Paridaens R, Jassem J, Delozier T, et al. A randomized trial of exemestane after two or three years of tamoxifen therapy in postmenopausal women with primary breast cancer. *N Engl J Med* 2004;350:1081–92.
- Early Breast Cancer Trialists' Collaborative Group. Tamoxifen for early breast cancer: an overview of the randomised trials. *Lancet* 1998;351:1451–67.
- Early Breast Cancer Trialists' Collaborative Group. Polychemotherapy for early breast cancer: an overview of the randomised trials. *Lancet* 1998;352:930–42.
- Eiermann W, Paepke S, Apffelstaedt J, Llombart-Cussac A, Eremin J, Vinholes J, et al. Preoperative treatment of postmenopausal breast cancer patients with letrozole: a randomized double-blind multicenter study. *Ann Oncol* 2001;12:1527–32.
- Ellis MJ, Coop A, Singh B, Maruriac L, Llombart-Cussac A, Janicke F, et al. Letrozole is more effective neoadjuvant endocrine therapy than tamoxifen for ErbB-1- and/or ErbB-2 positive, estrogen receptor-positive primary breast cancer: evidence from a phase III randomized trial. *J Clin Oncol* 2001;19:3808–16.
- Fisher B, Bryant J, Wolmark N, Mamoumas E, Brown A, Fisher ER, et al. Effect of preoperative chemotherapy on the outcome of women with operable breast cancer. *J Clin Oncol* 1998;16:2672–85
- Goss PE, Ingle JN, Martino S, Robert NJ, Muss HB, Piccart MJ, et al. A randomized trial of letrozole in postmenopausal women after five years of tamoxifen therapy for early-stage breast cancer. *N Engl J Med* 2003;349:1793–802.
- Henderson IC, Berry DA, Demetri GD, Cirrincione CT, Goldstein LJ, Murhio S, et al. Improved outcomes from adding sequential paclitaxel but not from escalating doxorubicin dose in an adjuvant chemotherapy regimen for patients with node-positive primary breast cancer. *J Clin Oncol* 2001;21:976–83.
- Powles T, Paterson S, Kanis J, McCloskey, Ashley J, Tidy A. Randomized, placebo-controlled trial of clodronate in patients with primary operable breast cancer. *J Clin Oncol* 2002;20:3219–24.
- Smith IE, Dowsett M. Aromatase inhibitors in breast cancer. *N Engl J Med* 2003;348:2431–42.

11 Locally advanced breast cancer

A Rodger, RCF Leonard, JM Dixon

Locally advanced disease of the breast is characterised clinically by features suggesting infiltration of the skin or chest wall by tumour or matted involved axillary nodes. Large operable breast cancers and tumours fixed to muscle should not be considered as locally advanced.

Locally advanced breast cancer may arise because of:
- the position in the breast (for example, peripheral or superficial)
- as a consequence of neglect (some patients do not present to hospital for months or years after they notice a mass). There is undoubtedly a major contribution from neglect as many cases arise in elderly patients in whom the cancers behave in a rather indolent manner and are often well controlled by endocrine therapy alone if surgery is not feasible due to general frailty
- biological aggressiveness (this includes all inflammatory cancers and most with peau d'orange). Inflammatory carcinomas are uncommon and are characterised by brawny, oedematous, indurated, and erythematous skin changes and have the worst prognosis of all locally advanced breast cancers.

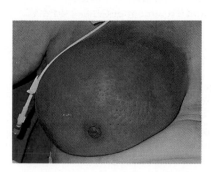
Inflammatory breast carcinoma

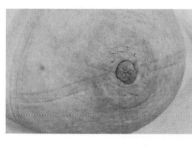
Peau d'orange associated with breast carcinoma

Clinical features of locally advanced breast cancer

Skin
- Ulceration
- Dermal infiltration
- Erythema over tumour
- Satellite nodules
- Peau d'orange

Axillary nodes
- Nodes fixed to one another or to other structures

Chest wall
Tumour fixation to:
- Ribs
- Serratus
- Intercostal muscle

Prognosis of locally advanced breast cancer

Recent data suggest that 5–10% of breast cancers present as locally advanced disease. Overall five year survival is about 50%, but prognosis relates to the biology of the underlying disease; indolent hormone sensitive disease does much better than hormone insensitive inflammatory breast cancer. Prognostic factors in locally advanced disease are similar to those in operable breast cancer: node status, tumour size, tumour biology including grade and proliferation rate, and response to treatment.

Treatment

Current treatments have increased local control of disease and have reduced the rate of metastatic progression. Despite changes in treatment, local and regional relapse remains a major problem and affects up to half of patients.

Role of systemic and local treatment

The mainstay of local treatment has been radiotherapy. This is because surgery, generally mastectomy, results in high rates of local recurrence. By contrast, though radiotherapy alone can produce high rates of local remission in both the breast and axilla, only 30% of patients remain free of locoregional disease at death. A sequence of appropriate systemic treatment and radiotherapy can increase the initial rate of local response to over 80%.

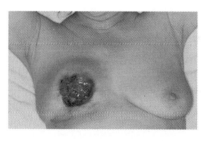
Ulcerated stage T$_4$ breast cancer

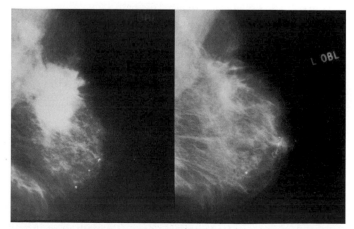
Mammogram of locally advanced breast tumour (left). Mammogram of same breast (right) after hormone therapy, showing substantial reduction in tumour volume (tumour was operable after treatment)

The aim of systemic treatment in this setting is to improve the chance of obtaining a complete and prolonged local remission and to increase survival. Most randomised controlled trials in true locally advanced disease have been of exceedingly poor quality. One major trial, however, (by the European Organisation for Research and Treatment of Cancer (EORTC)) has shown that while the addition of standard chemotherapy did not improve overall survival, the administration of appropriate hormone therapy to patients with hormone sensitive disease did.

If patients are fit, systemic therapy should be administered before local therapy with a view to reducing the extent of disease in the breast or axilla, or both. If the response is sufficient, surgery, mastectomy or breast conserving surgery if possible combined with axillary surgery, should be performed. This should then be followed by postmastectomy flap radiotherapy using a technique that includes the supraclavicular fossa (but avoiding the axilla if dissection has been performed).

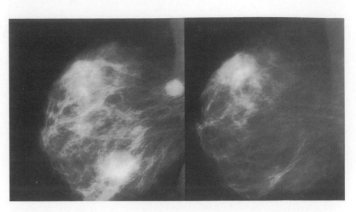

Stage T_4 cancer of the breast before (left) and after (right) chemotherapy, showing disappearance of mass lesion and axillary lymph node

Factors affecting choice of systemic treatment for locally advanced breast cancer

Hormonal treatment
- Slow growing or indolent disease
- Oestrogen receptor positive cancer
- Elderly or unfit patients

Chemotherapy
- Inflammatory cancer
- Oestrogen receptor negative cancer
- Rapidly progressive cancer

Choice of systemic treatment

Systemic treatment should be administered as part of a planned programme of combined systemic and local treatment. For frail patients treatment may initially be by endocrine therapy, with radiotherapy held in reserve for relapse.

Choice of systemic treatment for locally advanced breast cancer

Hormonal treatment
- Premenopausal women— ovarian ablation (surgery, radiation or gonadotrophin releasing hormone agents) plus tamoxifen*
- Postmenopausal women— letrozole*

Chemotherapy
- Intravenous anthracycline regimen[†] in combination with cyclophosphamide
- Intravenous taxane based regimen

Immunotherapy
- Trastuzumab in HER2 overexpression (3+ or 2+ and fluorescent in situ hybridization positive)

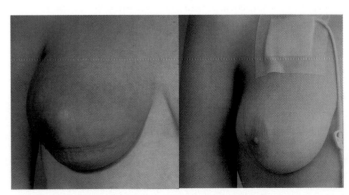

Locally advanced breast cancer (left) and complete clinical response after chemotherapy (right)

*Anastrozole and exemestane are other options
†For example, doxorubicin and cyclophosphamide or epirubicin and cyclophosphamide or taxane

Chemotherapy

Standard chemotherapy regimens have increased the initial rates of control. Studies of intensifying drug doses given in a fixed period either by giving smaller doses more frequently or by combining higher doses with factors to encourage regeneration of bone marrow does not produce survival benefits. Infusions of fluorouracil (F) combined with the anthracycline doxorubicin (A) and cisplatin (Cis) achieved a high overall response rate of 98% and a complete remission rate of over 60% in one pilot study, but a subsequent randomised trial comparing infusional ACisF with a combination of adriamycin and cyclophosphamide showed no significant difference in overall response rate, pathological complete remission, or five year survival. The role of taxanes in locally advanced breast cancer continues to be investigated.

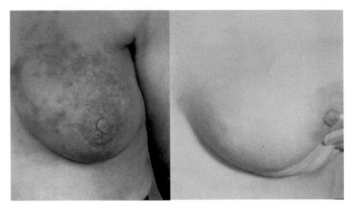

Inflammatory cancer of the breast before (left) and after (right) chemotherapy, showing an excellent response

Preliminary results have shown significantly higher rates of clinical response and pathological complete remission with the addition of docetaxel to adriamycin and cyclophosphamide. Two studies have shown that patients responding to four courses of anthracycline based chemotherapy and subsequently randomised to four further courses of docetaxel had a higher overall rate of response and pathological remission than those receiving four further cycles of the same chemotherapy. Updated NSABP results have shown a reduction in local recurrence with the addition of docetaxel, but no improvement in survival. All the trials included patients with large operable breast cancer, and some included patients with locally advanced breast cancer. Not all trials have shown a benefit from adding taxanes; a UK study that included patients with large operable and locally advanced breast cancer found that the response rate to the combination of adriamycin and docetaxel was identical to that obtained with adriamycin and cyclophosphamide.

Early reports of trials investigating the role of trastuzumab in patients whose tumours express the erbB2 or HER2 oncogene product have been encouraging, with higher response rates for patients treated with neoadjuvant chemotherapy and trastuzumab together than for patients treated with neoadjuvant chemotherapy alone.

As data from trials mature it may be possible to obtain better initial clinical and radiological responses, enabling more patients to become suitable for surgery and radiotherapy. Increasing response rates and improving the quality of the responses should improve long term local control and may also delay metastatic relapse and improve survival.

Hormonal therapy

An EORTC study has shown that hormonal therapy plays an important part in reducing the risk of locoregional failure, distant metastases, and mortality in patients with hormone receptor positive disease. Substantial reductions in tumour volume with endocrine therapy alone can be achieved in patients with tumours with high levels of oestrogen receptor. The newer aromatase inhibitors are superior to tamoxifen in postmenopausal women. Drugs such as letrozole can also be effective, even in inflammatory cancers providing the tumour is oestrogen receptor rich.

Radiotherapy

Radiotherapy is generally well tolerated, even by elderly and frail patients. It can be given concurrently with systemic hormonal treatment or after a course of primary chemotherapy. The breast skin requires full dose, and this will result in temporary erythema and probable moist desquamation. If possible, palpable tumour masses should receive treatment boosts with either electrons or interstitial brachytherapy. Such

Radiotherapy for locally advanced breast cancer

Treatment areas
- Breast
- Axilla and supraclavicular fossa (the axilla should be omitted if the patient has had a complete axillary dissection)

Treatment
- Megavoltage x rays
- Technique for enhancing skin dose
- 40–50 Gy in 15–25 fractions over 3–5 weeks
- Boost to tumour mass if possible by external beam or radioactive implant of 10–20 Gy

Toxicity
- Lethargy
- Skin erythema and areas of moist desquamation
- Temporary mild dysphagia
- Less than 1% risk of pneumonitis

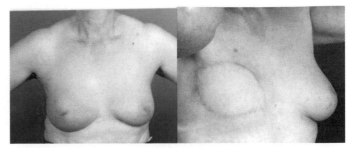

Stage T$_4$ cancer of the breast before (left) and after (right) chemotherapy, radiotherapy, and surgery

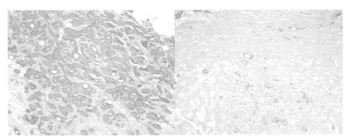

Invasive ductal carcinoma before (left) and after chemotherapy (right), showing extensive hyaline fibrosis and reduction in tumour bulk

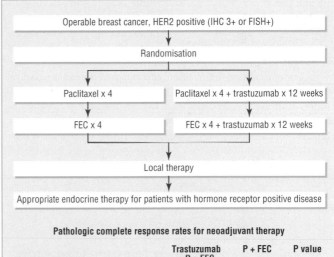

| Operable breast cancer, HER2 positive (IHC 3+ or FISH+) |
| Randomisation |
| Paclitaxel x 4 | Paclitaxel x 4 + trastuzumab x 12 weeks |
| FEC x 4 | FEC x 4 + trastuzumab x 12 weeks |
| Local therapy |
| Appropriate endocrine therapy for patients with hormone receptor positive disease |

Pathologic complete response rates for neoadjuvant therapy

	Trastuzumab + P + FEC	P + FEC	P value
Overall (n=2319)	65.2%	26.3%	0.016
Hormone receptor-positive (n=1311)	61.5%	27.2%	-
Hormone receptor-negative (n=108)	70.0%	25.0%	-

MD Anderson randomised trial of neoadjuvant trastuzumab and chemotherapy. (FEC = fluorouracil, epirubicin and cyclophosphamide, FISH = fluorescent in situ hybridisation, IHC = immunohistochemistry, P = paclitaxel). Adapted from Buzdar AU et al. presentation at ASCO, 2004

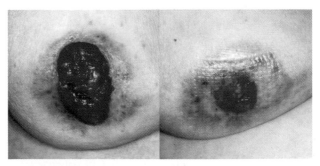

Locally advanced breast cancer before (left) and after three months of treatment with letrozole (right). This patient was treated with breast conserving surgery and radiotherapy

boosts should be considered for palpable disease in the breast or axilla, or both. For particularly refractory tumours, radiotherapy is sometimes given concurrently with radiosensitising chemotherapy agents such as 5 fluorouracil.

Surgery

Mastectomy is generally not possible in the presence of features of locally advanced disease, but the role of surgery is changing. Intensive treatment with a combination of cytotoxic drugs or initial hormonal treatment often causes the primary tumour to regress to a lower stage (with disappearance of peau d'orange and erythema and reduction in tumour volume), making surgery feasible some weeks or months after the start of systemic treatment. In such cases surgery may be a wide excision and sentinel node biopsy or clearance of axillary nodes but is more usually a total mastectomy and node clearance, both being followed by radiotherapy to the remaining breast or the chest wall.

Breast conservation is possible in patients whose tumours have reduced in size with systemic therapy. Wide excision after hormone therapy is usually successful, with clear margins being obtained; in contrast, after neoadjuvant chemotherapy in some patients multiple residual islands of tumour are sometimes seen, requiring re-excision or mastectomy to ensure complete excision of all remaining disease.

Management of residual disease

In some patients residual disease remains in the breast despite systemic treatment and radiotherapy. The disease can be excised by a salvage mastectomy, ideally followed by coverage with a myocutaneous flap (latissimus dorsi or transverse rectus abdominus). "Toilet" surgery, used in an effort to control fungating cancers or recurrence and progression of disease, is often ineffective and should be performed only for breast cancers that are locally advanced, either because of their peripheral position in the breast or because of a delay in presentation. In this group surgery should be combined with radiotherapy and appropriate adjuvant systemic treatment.

Despite the best efforts with combined treatments, a substantial proportion of patients who present with locally advanced disease develop uncontrolled disease of the chest wall. Although chemotherapy can relieve symptoms in up to half of these patients, the overall efficacy of systemic chemotherapy is poor.

Recently, other cytotoxic agents have been shown to have an effect in locally recurrent and locally advanced breast cancer. Thus third and even fourth lines of chemotherapy, using, for example, the oral agent capecitabine or intravenous vinorelbine, are sometimes effective in patients with these intractable and unpleasant conditions.

Rarely, retreatment with radiotherapy is possible using brachytherapy with radioactive sources applied to the surface or superficial x rays. An alternative may be local hyperthermia, which is available in a few centres.

Patients with hormone sensitive disease may experience temporary responses from a change in hormone therapy using, in sequence, aromatase inhibitors, antioestrogens (tamoxifen or fulvestrant or both), progestogens, and even oestrogens.

Local recurrence after mastectomy

This usually occurs in the skin flaps adjacent to the scar and is presumed to arise from viable cells shed during surgery. It can be diagnosed by fine needle aspiration cytology or core biopsy. Local disease can be isolated, but in up to half of patients it heralds systemic relapse. For this reason a search for distant metastases should be undertaken in all patients.

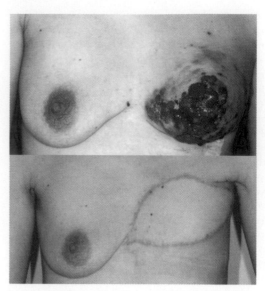

Patient who had previously been treated with radiotherapy for Hodgkin's disease with a locally advanced breast cancer before (top) and after (bottom) a latissimus dorsi flap for chest wall cover. The disease had originally responded to chemotherapy but then progressed

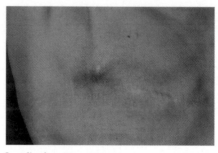

Localised spot recurrence

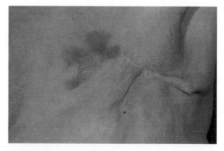

Multiple spot recurrence

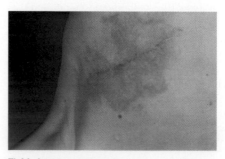

Field change recurrence

Local recurrence after mastectomy can be classified as single spot relapse, multiple spot relapse, or field change. Treatment differs for these three categories, as does prognosis with the worse survival in those with field change.

Treatment

If the recurrence is focal and occurs many years after the original surgery, excision alone can provide long term control. If the recurrence is focal but occurs within the first few years after mastectomy then excision should be combined with radiotherapy if not previously given. If the recurrence is not single but still localised then the options are radiotherapy or more radical excision followed by radiotherapy. A change in systemic therapy should also be considered for patients with localised or multiple spot recurrence. In more widespread recurrence the standard treatments are often disappointing. Radiotherapy at a high skin dose should be considered if it has not been given before. Failure to halt the progress of local disease can lead to cancer en cuirasse—in which the chest wall is encircled by tumour—an extremely unpleasant situation for the patient. Systemic therapies used for this are the same as for the management of residual disease above.

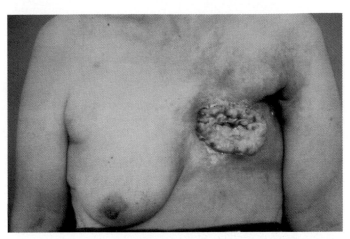

Longstanding, isolated, large, unsightly, and malodorous local recurrence after mastectomy and radiotherapy

---

Treatment of local recurrence in chest wall

Single spot

- Excise and consider radiotherapy—consider hormonal treatment if tumour is oestrogen receptor positive

Multiple spot

- Radiotherapy, unless already given, or more radical excision (possible with coverage with myocutaneous flap); consider change in systemic treatment

Widespread

- Consider radiotherapy, unless already given or disease too widespread
- Give appropriate systemic therapy (hormonal or chemotherapy) depending on oestrogen receptor and disease behaviour
- Consider oral capecitabine

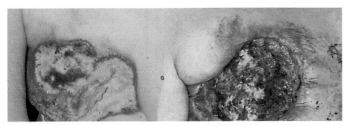

Ulcerated breast cancer before (left) and after (right) debridement

Recurrence on the chest wall can sometimes be quite indolent, and slowly growing, and can occur in the absence of metastases elsewhere. Multiple small spot recurrences of ≤1 cm in the dermis may respond for several months to topical cytotoxic agents such as miltefosine. The control of ulceration and focal malodorous infected tissue is a considerable problem for carers, and patients with such disease have a miserable existence. Excision of dead tissue and the use of topical and oral antibiotics with antianaerobic activity combined with charcoal dressings can help to control the odour. The best form of treatment is prevention by ensuring that initial local treatment is optimal.

Further reading

- Bear HD, Anderson S, Brown A, Smith R, Mamounas EP, Fisher B, et al. The effect on tumor response of adding sequential preoperative docetaxel to preoperative doxorubicin and cyclophosphamide: preliminary results from national surgical adjuvant breast and bowel project protocol B-27. *J Clin Oncol* 2003;21:4165–74.
- von Minckwitz G, Raab G, Schuette M, Hilfrisch J, Blohmer JM, Gerber B, et al. Dose-dense versus sequential adriamycin/docetaxel combination as preoperative chemotherapy (pCHT) in operable breast cancer (T2–3, N0–2,M0)—primary endpoint analysis of the GePARDUO Study. *Proc Am Soc Oncol* 2002;21:43a.
- Smith IC, Heys SD, Hutcheon AW, Miller ID, Payne S, Gilbert FJ, et al. Neoadjuvant chemotherapy in breast cancer: significantly enhanced response with docetaxel. *J Clin Oncol* 2002;20:1456–66.

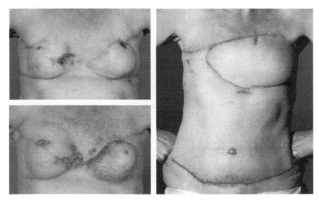

Patient with bilateral breast reconstructions (latissimus dorsi flap for left breast, implant and expander for right breast) who developed chest wall recurrence (top left) that was initially retreated with radiotherapy (bottom left) and then excision and a free transverse rectus abdominus myocutaneous flap (right)

12 Metastatic breast cancer

RCF Leonard, A Rodger, JM Dixon

When cancers metastasise, few other cancers have such a variable natural course and effect on survival as breast cancer. Patients with hormone sensitive cancers may live for several years without any intervention other than various sequential hormonal manipulations. In contrast, patients with disease that is not sensitive to hormones have a much shorter interval free of disease and shorter survival, reflecting the more aggressive biology of hormone independent cancers. The average period of survival after diagnosis of metastatic disease is 18–24 months, but this varies between patients.

Clinical patterns of relapse predict future behaviour. Patients with a long interval without disease after primary diagnosis (more than two years) and favourable sites of recurrence (such as local lymph nodes and the chest wall) survive longer than patients with a short interval without disease or recurrence at other sites. Patients with visceral disease have the poorest outlook; these patients tend to have a short interval without disease and cancers that are biologically more aggressive.

Treatment of metastatic disease

A patient may present with metastatic breast carcinoma or develop a systemic recurrence after treatment for an apparently localised breast cancer. The aim of treatment is to control the symptoms with minimal side effects. In terms of drug treatment this ideal is achieved only by hormonal treatment in the 30% of patients whose cancers respond to such drugs. There is no evidence that treating patients with asymptomatic metastases improves overall survival, and chemotherapy should be given routinely to symptomatic patients only.

Hormonal treatment

A variety of hormonal drugs is available for use in metastatic breast cancer. Objective responses to hormonal treatment are seen in 30% of all patients and in 50–60% of patients with oestrogen receptor positive tumours. Response rates of 25% are seen with second line hormonal treatments, although less than 15% of patients who show no response to first line hormonal treatment will respond to second line treatment, and 10–15% respond to third line treatment.

Premenopausal women
A combination of tamoxifen and goserelin is superior to either drug alone. Current studies are comparing this combination with goserelin and an aromatase inhibitor.

Postmenopausal women
Until recently tamoxifen was the most commonly prescribed drug in postmenopausal women who had not received it as adjuvant treatment. The advent of third generation aromatase inhibitors has changed this. Results from large randomised trials that compared tamoxifen and anastrozole, letrozole and exemestane showed that these drugs are well tolerated and more effective than tamoxifen. An analysis of North American and European studies that compared anastrozole with tamoxifen in the first line metastatic setting showed a superior time to progression in patients with oestrogen receptor positive breast cancer in patients treated with anastrozole. A large study that compared letrozole with tamoxifen showed letrozole to be

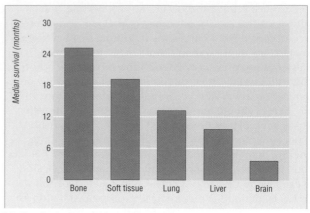

Median time of survival associated with sites of metastasis in patients with breast cancer

Endocrine drugs for breast cancer

Antioestrogens
- Tamoxifen
- Toremifene
- Fulvestrant

Aromatase inhibitors
- Anastrozole
- Letrozole
- Exemestane

Progestins
- Megestrol acetate
- Medroxyprogesterone acetate

Oestrogens
- Estrodiol
- Diethylstilbestrol

Androgens
- Fluoxymesterone

Luteinising hormone releasing hormone analogues
- Goserelin
- Leuprolide
- Buserelin

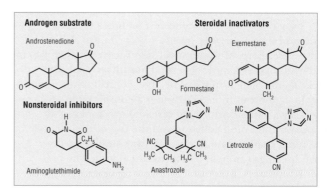

Structures of antiaromatase drugs

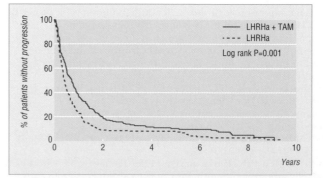

Meta analysis of trials in premenopausal women with metastatic breast cancer comparing luteinising releasing hormone analogues (LHRHa) with or without tamoxifen (TAM): progression free survival. Adapted from Klijn JG et al. *J Clin Oncol* 2001;19:343–53

superior in all outcomes in all groups of patients, with a superior response rate (31% v 21%), and a longer time to progression and treatment failure, prolonged time to chemotherapy, and a substantially better survival profile in the first two years of treatment. A study comparing exemestane and tamoxifen showed a significantly greater response rate with exemestane (46%) compared with tamoxifen (31%), but no significant difference in progression free or overall survival. Letrozole or anastrozole are the drugs of choice for patients with oestrogen receptor positive metastatic breast cancer who have previously received adjuvant tamoxifen.

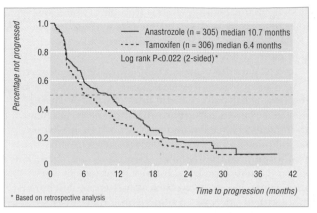

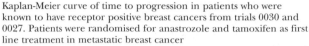

Kaplan-Meier curve of time to progression in patients who were known to have receptor positive breast cancers from trials 0030 and 0027. Patients were randomised for anastrozole and tamoxifen as first line treatment in metastatic breast cancer

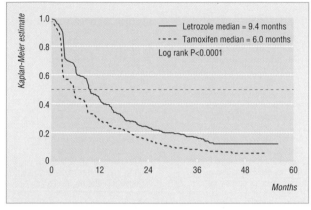

Kaplan-Meier curve of time to treatment progression in first line randomised study of letrozole or tamoxifen in patients with metastatic breast cancer. From *J Clin Oncol* 2003;21:2101–9

After failure of the non-steroidal aromatase inhibitors letrozole or anastrozole, the choice of drugs includes tamoxifen (if not used previously), exemestane (a steroidal aromatase inactivator), and fulvestrant. Approximately one quarter of these patients will get clinical benefit with exemestane. Having a novel mechanism of action, fulvestrant downregulates oestrogen receptor expression. Given as an intramuscular injection once a month it has been compared with anastrozole in the second line setting, and with tamoxifen as first line treatment. Fulvestrant is as effective as either anastrozole or tamoxifen in patients with oestrogen receptor positive cancer. The progestogens, megestrol acetate and medroxyprogesterone, are still used occasionally as third or fourth line drugs. Although they are effective, they have been superceded by newer drugs with a better side effect profile.

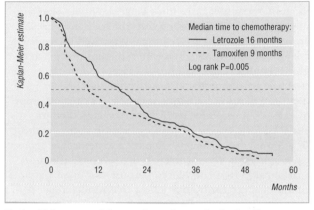

Kaplan-Meier curve of time to chemotherapy in the first line randomised study of letrozole or tamoxifen in patients with metastatic breast cancer. From *J Clin Oncol* 2003; 21: 2101–9

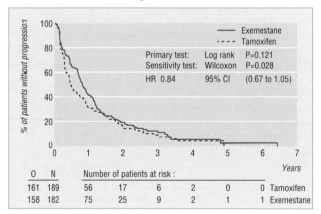

Kaplan-Meier curve for time to treatment progression from the phase II randomised trial of first line hormonal treatment with exemestane or tamoxifen in postmenopausal women with metastatic breast cancer (presented at ASCO 2004)

Response to exemestane after failure of second line aromatase inhibitors*

	Prior aromatase inhibitors		
	Aminogluteth-imide (n = 136)	Non-steroidal aromatase inhibitor (n = 105)	All aromatase inhibitors (n = 241)
Complete remission	2 (1.5%)	1 (1.0%)	3 (1.2%)
Partial remission	9 (6.6%)	4 (3.8%)	13 (5.4%)
Overall response rate	11 (8.1%)	5 (4.8%)	16 (6.6%)
SD > 6 months	26 (19.1%)	16 (15.2%)	42 (17.4%)
Clinical benefit	37 (27.2%)	21 (20.0%)	58 (24.0%)

* Adapted from Lønning, PE et al. *J Clin Oncol* 2000;18:2234–44

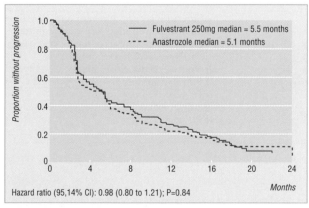

Time to progression curves from the European phase III trial of fulvestrant versus anastrozole in the second line setting (after tamoxifen) in patients with metastatic breast cancer

One drug that is being revived is trilostane, which was developed mistakenly as a weak aromatase inhibitor in the early 1990s. New research shows that it inhibits the classical oestrogen pathway, but also blocks a second pathway mediated by AP-1 and may mediate growth inhibition after "oestrogen escape" irrespective of menopausal status. The persistence of good response activity after several lines of prior endocrine treatment in earlier trials supports this hypothesis, but new trials are underway after the failure of aromatase inhibitors.

After cells develop resistance to antioestrogens and oestrogen withdrawal they become sensitive to oestrogen. This observation has led to renewed interest in using pharmacological doses of oestrogen. Patients can develop an initial flare with an increase in bone pain if metastases are present, but impressive and long lasting responses are seen with oestrogen in some patients.

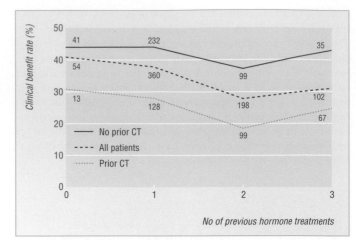

Clinical benefit rate with trilostane in heavily pretreated postmenopausal patients with advanced breast cancer (n = 714) (CT = chemotherapy)

Chemotherapy

With chemotherapy, a balance must be achieved between a high rate of response and limiting side effects. Randomised trials showed that more active regimens improved survival. The best palliation is usually obtained with regimens that produce the highest response rates. Overall rates of response to chemotherapy are about 40–60%, with a median time to relapse of 6–10 months. Subsequent courses of chemotherapy have lower rates of response (<25%). The chemotherapy regimens used for metastatic breast cancer are similar to those used for adjuvant and primary systemic treatment. Analogues of the most potent drug (doxorubicin) such as epirubicin and mitoxantrone are often considered because they have a greater safety margin for the cardiotoxic effect that results from continued exposure.

Which cytotoxics are effective?

Many drugs are effective and active in the treatment of metastatic breast cancer. Taxanes are effective in disease resistant to anthracyclines (response rate of 30–40%), and they are the most commonly used drugs after relapse in women exposed to anthracyclines. They are used for metastatic disease or in the adjuvant setting. The activity of docetaxel given every three weeks is greater than that of paclitaxel, but side effects and morbidity are greater with docetaxel. Giving paclitaxel weekly seems to increase efficacy without increasing side effects; a study to compare a weekly and three weekly regimens is ongoing.

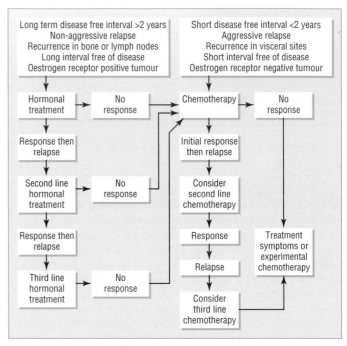

Selection for treatment of metastatic or recurrent breast cancer

Common regimens for metastatic breast cancer

Regimen	Efficacy (% response)	Toxicity	Comments
AC/EC/FAC/FEC*	40–50	m++;a++;c+;n++	Not useful if recent adjuvant anthracyclines
Docetaxel*	35–45	m+++;a+;n+;ne++	Use if anthracycline in adjuvant regimen
Paclitaxel*	25–35	m++;a++;n+;ne+++	Use if anthracycline in adjuvant regimen
Paclitaxel/gemcitabine*	40	m++;a++;n+;ne+++	Alternative to paclitaxel alone
Docetaxel/capecitabine*	50–60	m++;a+;n++;ne++;hfd++	Alternative to docetaxel alone
Taxane/Trastuzumab*	50–60	As above plus cardiotoxicity	HER2 positive only
Trastuzumab†	20–30	Cardiotoxicity only	HER2 positive only
Vinorelbine†	20–30	m++;a+;n+;ne++	Usually after taxane failure
Vinorelbine/trastuzumab†	50–60	m++;a+;n+;ne++;c+	HER2 positive only
Capecitabine†	30	m+;hfd++	Usually after taxane failure

*Usually first relapse setting

†Usually second or third relapse setting

(A = adriamycin, C = cyclophosphamide, E = epirubicin, F = fluorouracil)

Toxicity is as follows: a = alopecia, c = cardiotoxicity, hfd = hand and foot syndrome and diarrhoea, m = myelosuppression, n = nausea and vomiting, ne = neurotoxicity

In the presence of bone disease, bisphosphonates are often used alone or concurrently with chemotherapy or endocrine therapy to improve control of bone complications. Intravenous or oral bisphosphonates are used for up to two years

Taxanes have largely displaced other second and third line regimens such as vinblastine and mitomycin C. The vinca alkaloid, vinorelbine, is well tolerated and has activity as second line therapy, either alone or in combination. An orally active fluoropyrimidine, capecitabine, mimics the pharmacology of continuously infused intravenous 5-fluorouracil. One phase III trial compared the combination of capecitabine and docetaxel (the latter at 25% dose reduction) in matched patient groups as first, second, or third line chemotherapy with the most potent single drug (docetaxel) at 100% dose. The combination produced a superior response rate and better survival. Data now support the view that the most active chemotherapy regimens produce clinically useful survival gains for patients. This is an important development in care.

Bisphosphonates

Bisphosphonates are an established part of the routine treatment of widespread bony disease. Randomised trials have shown that bisphosphonates reduce the need for radiotherapy and reduce symptomatic complications of patients with metastatic bone disease. Bisphosphonates are given as infusions or orally every month, although their relatively poor bioavailability reduces absorption. Intravenous pamidronate was the most commonly used drug, but now zoledronate, a new potent bisphosphonate, has become the intravenous bisphosphonate of choice as it reduces skeletal morbidity compared with pamidronate, and can be given as a 15 minute infusion rather than the two hours needed for pamidronate. Ibandronate is a potent oral drug. Trials to compare it with zoledronate are underway. Guidelines are used to identify those patients who benefit most from these drugs.

Immunotherapy

Between 25% and 30% of breast cancers overexpress the oncoproteins HER2-neu or erbB2. The humanised murine antibody trastuzumab has antitumour activity against cells that overexpress HER2. Phase I and phase II clinical trials have shown that multiple doses of antibody can be given safely. The results of large randomised trials have shown that trastuzumab is effective as a single agent, but it may act synergistically with chemotherapeutic drugs. Patients with breast cancer refractory to doxorubicin treated with trastuzumab and paclitaxel in one study had almost double the response rate and improvements in time to progression and survival compared with those given paclitaxel alone. As a result of this study and others, trastuzumab is now standard care given alone or in combination with taxanes in patients with advanced cancers that overexpress HER2. Trastuzumab treatment should continue until resistance to treatment is apparent. Although the pivotal trial data relate to paclitaxel, trastuzumab is often given in combination with the most active of the taxanes, docetaxel. This combination is well tolerated, but there is a risk of cardiac failure.

Specific problems

Sites of relapse and their management

Bone disease

The bony skeleton is a site of relapse in three quarters of patients who develop secondary breast cancer. Diagnosis is usually possible by bone scan or plain x rays or both. Magnetic resonance imaging is more sensitive and is indicated where scans are equivocal or where bone metastases are considered likely, but other tests have been negative. Computed tomography scans can also visualise bony destruction. Widespread bone disease often responds well to hormonal

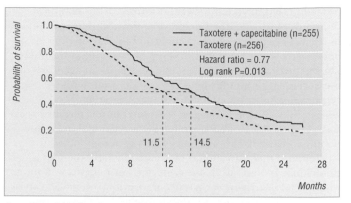

Overall survival of patients with metastatic breast cancer randomised to receive taxotere alone or a combination of capecitabine and taxotere. From O'Shaughnessy J et al. *J Clin Oncol* 2002;20:2812–23

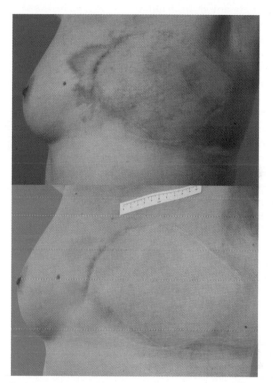

Patient with inflammatory type local recurrence three years after mastectomy and latissimus dorsi flap before start of treatment (top). The cancer was HER2 3+ on testing and the patient was treated with six cycles of taxotere and three weekly trastuzumab. The patient continued on three weekly trastuzumab and no disease was visible 18 months later (bottom)

Results from trials with trastuzumab in patients with metastatic breast cancer whose tumours overexpressed HER2 and who received first line treatment with chemotherapy alone or chemotherapy with trastuzumab*

	Objective response rate	Time to progresssion	Overall survival (months)
Chemotherapy	32%	4.6	20.3
Chemotherapy and trastuzumab	50%	7.4	25.1
P value	<0.001	<0.001	0.025
Paclitaxel alone	15%	3.0	18.4
Paclitaxel and trastuzumab	42%	6.9	22.1
P value	<0.001	<0.001	Not significant

*Adapted from *N Engl J Med* 2001;344:783–92

treatment, but in young patients cytotoxic drugs may be required. Measuring the benefit of anticancer drug treatment in terms of objective regression of tumour may be difficult, as bone scans are unreliable indicators of response to treatment. For this reason, repeated magnetic resonance image scans or measurement of tumour markers is often used to assess response in bony metastatic disease. Collagen markers (N telopeptides of type I collagen cross links and C terminal cross linked telopeptide of collagen type I) are being evaluated as potential markers of bone activity and treatment efficacy.

Localised bone pain should be treated by radiotherapy: a single dose is often all that is required. For patients with more widespread disease or recurrence in previously irradiated areas, alternative measures are required. Analgesic drugs are the mainstay of treatment, either as a prelude to effective anticancer treatment or as a long term alternative or supplement to this treatment. Non-steroidal anti-inflammatory drugs are surprisingly potent in dealing with bone pain, even compared with opiates. Combining the two classes of drugs increases efficacy while minimising side effects.

Widespread bone pain may also be treated by simple analgesia combined with radiotherapy and bisphosphonates.

Pathological fractures caused by bone metastases should be avoided and can be predicted by a sharp increase in pain over a few days or weeks. When bone lysis threatens fracture, internal fixation followed by radiotherapy (low dose in a few fractions) will improve quality of life and mobility and can be associated with a reasonable survival. If a pathological fracture does occur, the same combination of internal fixation and radiotherapy is used, but the functional result is inferior to that of prophylactic treatment.

Treatment of bone metastases

Consider bisphosphonates

Localised bone pain
- External beam radiotherapy
- Analgesics including opiates
- Non-steroidal anti-inflammatory drugs

Widespread bone pain
- Radioactive strontium
- Sequential hemibody radiotherapy
- Analgesics including opiates
- Non-steroidal anti-inflammatory drugs

Pathological fractures*
- Internal fixation and radiotherapy

---

*Also prophylactic treatment for patients at risk of fracture

Marrow infiltration

Any of the peripheral blood elements may be reduced by marrow infiltration, but a "leukoerythroblastic picture" (immature cells in the peripheral blood) suggests extensive marrow infiltration. Chemotherapy is generally used and should be given initially in reduced doses, with careful monitoring and adequate supportive care. A weekly regimen of bolus epirubicin or doxorubicin ($25–30 \text{ mg/m}^2$) or weekly paclitaxel ($80–90 \text{ mg/m}^2$) is well tolerated and effective. In hormone receptor positive disease, excellent and long lived responses are seen with endocrine therapy even with substantial bone marrow infiltration.

Malignant pleural effusion

Up to half of patients with metastatic breast cancer will develop a malignant pleural effusion, but only some of these will require specific treatment. Cytological examination of effusion fluid is positive for malignant cells in around 85% of patients. Aspiration of fluid alone is ineffective in controlling malignant

Scoring system for long term bisphosphate treatment for metastatic breast cancer—total score for a patient is calculated and aids selection of patients who should receive long term bisphosphate treatment

Extent of disease	Score
Bone (marrow)only	3
Bone and soft tissue	2
Bone and visceral disease	1
Bone morbidity	
Previous skeletal even with or without bone pain	3
Bone pain	2
Asymptomatic	1
Eastern Co-operative Oncology Group (ECOG) performance status:	
1,2	3
0,3	2
4	1
Underlying treatment:	
Needing chemotherapy or endocrine resistance	2
Potentially endocrine resistant	1
Good prognosis factors:	
Disease free interval >3 years	1
Ductal grade 1 or 2 lobular history	
Bone metastases at initial presentation	

Total score and interpretation
Total score: >11: high priority for long term bisphosphate treatment
7–11: moderate priority for long term bisphosphate treatment
<7 Low priority for long term bisphosphate treatment

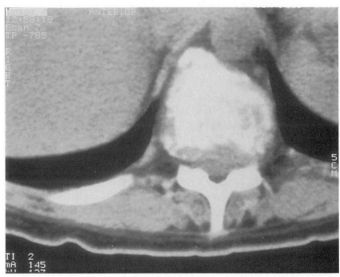

Computed tomography scan of lumbar vertebrae showing involvement by metastatic breast cancer

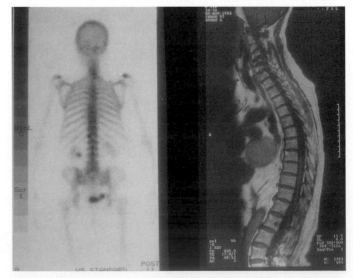

Bone scan showing a normal skeleton but a magnetic resonance image scan showed a lumbar vertebral involvement by metastatic breast cancer

pleural effusions, and 97–100% of patients reaccumulate fluid. By contrast, tube drainage alone is effective in controlling effusions in just over a third of patients. For the remaining patients, installation of bleomycin, tetracycline, talc, or inactivated *Corynebacterium parvum* is required to control recurrence. All are relatively safe, and the main problems are pain (usually transient) and pyrexia.

Malignant hypercalcaemia

This is a potentially fatal complication. The onset is often insidious, and it may present as a non-specific illness and general deterioration of health leading to confusion, dehydration, renal failure, and coma. The treatment of this complication has been transformed by the availability of bisphosphonates, and these are the drugs of choice after hydration with saline (about 3 l given over 24 hours). Effective anticancer treatment reduces the risk of recurrence, but patients whose disease is refractory to this treatment and who exhibit continuing hypercalcaemia can be treated with intravenous bisphosphonates given every two to four weeks.

Neurological complications

Although non-metastatic syndromes of the central nervous system can occur with breast cancer, any focal neurological symptom must be investigated. Computed tomography or better, magnetic resonance imaging can detect even small volumes of disease in the brain. Isotope brain scanning is unhelpful. Cord disease is best detected by magnetic resonance imaging. The initial treatment of brain metastases is to reduce oedema with high dose corticosteroids (16 mg daily of dexamethasone), pending local treatment with fractionated radiotherapy. Radiotherapy produces most benefit in patients whose neurological symptoms improve after taking steroids. Radiotherapy may be given in 5–10 fractions.

Long term survival may occur in patients with a solitary brain metastasis if no evidence of involvement of visceral sites is present and the disease is hormone responsive. Isolated disease at a favourable site in the brain is best treated by excision of the metastasis followed by postoperative radiotherapy or by stereotactic radiosurgery and whole brain radiotherapy, and appropriate systemic treatment.

Cord compression is not usually amenable to surgery and is seen most often in patients with thoracic spinal metastases. Treatment with steroids and fractionated radiotherapy (5–10 treatments) may produce dramatic responses provided that treatment is started as soon as possible before neurological deficits (paraparesis and bladder and bowel dysfunction) are severe. Patients with isolated metastases that cause cord compression who are fit can be treated by emergency laminectomy. Occasionally patients develop meningeal infiltration, which can result in cranial nerve damage. Treatment by drugs (intrathecal methotrexate) or radiotherapy, or both, can be effective. Infiltration or compression of nerves (such as infiltration of the brachial plexus) by a tumour can produce pain, paresis, and paraesthesia. Palliative radiotherapy helps but analgesic drugs, often in combination with drugs such as carbamazepine, amitriptyline, or mexiletine, may be required.

Control of pain

Most patients with metastatic breast cancer complain of pain at some stage of their illness. These patients rarely have one site of pain, and most have several pains that may have different causes. Each site of pain and the mechanism underlying the pain should be identified. Patients' emotional states (anger, despair, fear, anxiety, or depression) may be important in

Treatment of hypercalcaemia in breast cancer

- Hydration
- Bisphosphonates
- Mobilisation
- Anticancer treatment

> The long term results of treating disease of the central nervous system are disappointing, with most patients dying within three to four months

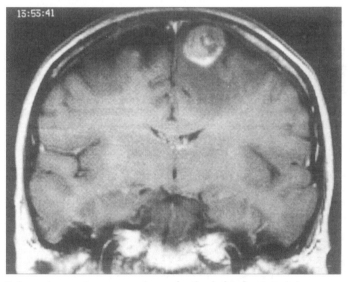

Enhanced magnetic resonance image showing isolated metastasis in frontoparietal region. In the absence of any other disease, this is suitable for treatment by excision and postoperative radiotherapy

Choice of analgesic for control of pain

Pain	Class of analgesic	Preferred drug
Mild	Simple analgesic	Paracetamol (preferable to aspirin because of lack of gastrointestinal side effects)
Moderate	Weak opioid analgesic (alone or in combination with simple analgesic)	Codeine with paracetamol
Severe	Strong opioid analgesic	Morphine

relation to how they respond to their pain and need to be assessed and treated as part of their pain.

Analgesia should be simple, flexible, and appropriate for the severity of the pain. If simple or weak opioid analgesics do not bring the pain under control quickly, treatment with strong opioid analgesics or adjuvant drugs should be started. Laxatives should be given to patients treated with opiates to prevent constipation. Some drugs have no intrinsic analgesic activity but can contribute significantly to pain control when used in combination with analgesics. Anxiety, restlessness, and insomnia may be treated with benzodiazepines. The place of antidepressants in the management of chronic pain is not clear, but some patients with advanced or terminal malignant disease do seem to respond to them.

Patients with breast cancer can also have other symptoms that require treatment, including anorexia, dysphagia, nausea and vomiting, respiratory symptoms, headache, and malodorous ulceration of the chest wall.

Although it may not be possible to cure or prolong the lives of some patients with metastatic breast cancer, much can be done to improve their quality of life. Management of cancer patients with end stage disease should be multidisciplinary and should involve palliative care physicians or physicians with an interest in treating pain. Control of symptoms is only one aspect of palliative care, and the resources of a skilled multidisciplinary team are needed to ensure that the psychological and social problems of patients and their families are dealt with in the most appropriate way.

Adjuvant drugs for control of pain

Cause of pain	Useful adjuvant drug
Soft tissue infiltration	Non-steroidal anti-inflammatory drugs Prednisolone*
Bone pain	Non-steroidal anti-inflammatory drugs
Hepatic enlargement	Prednisolone
Raised intracranial pressure	Dexamethasone†
Compression or infiltration of nerves	Dexamethasone†
(Dysaesthetic pain)	Carbamazepine Mexiletine
Muscle spasm	Diazepam Baclofen
Fungating tumour	Antibiotics Systemic co-amoxiclav or metronidazole Topical metronidazole
Cellulitis	Systemic antibiotics

*30–40 mg daily; withdraw if no effect in two weeks

†Initial dose of 12–16 mg daily, gradually reducing dose to minimum needed for control of symptoms

Control of other symptoms with metastatic breast cancer

Symptom	Treatment
Anorexia	Prednisolone or progestogens
Dysphagia	Antifungal drugs if related to candidiasis External beam irradiation, surgical intubation, or endoscopic laser treatment if mechanical evidence of obstruction Consider chemotherapy if dysphagia results from mediastinal node compression
Nausea and vomiting	Treat underlying cause Antiemetics (such as metoclopramide or cyclizine) with or without prednisolone
Constipation	Laxative
Dyspnoea	Morphine and benzodiazepines
Cough	Codeine or methadone linctus or morphine oral solution Nebulised local anaesthetics

Further reading

- Chan S, Friedrichs K, Noel D, Duarte R, Pinter T, Van Belle S, Vorobiof D, et al. Prospective randomised trial of doxatel versus doxorubicin in patients with metastatic breast cancer. *J Clin Oncol* 1999;17:2341–54.
- Greenberg AC, Hortobagyi GN, Smith TL, Ziegler LD, Frye DK, Buzdar AU. Long-term follow-up of patients with complete remission following combination chemotherapy for metastatic breast cancer. *J Clin Oncol* 1997;14:2197–205.
- Mouridsen H, Gershanovich M, Sun Y, Perez-Carrion R, Boni C, Monnier A, et al. Phase III study of letrozole versus tamoxifen as first-line therapy of advanced breast cancer in postmenopausal women: analysis of survival and update of efficacy from the International Letrozole Breast Cancer Group. *J Clin Oncol* 2003;21:2101–9.
- Thurlimann B, Robertson JF, Nabholtz JM, Buzdar A, Bonneterre J for the Arimidex Study Group. Efficacy of tamoxifen following anastrozole ('Arimidex') compared with anastrozole following tamoxifen as first-line treatment for advanced breast cancer in postmenopausal women. *Eur J Cancer* 2003;39:2310–17.
- Slamon DJ, Leyland-Jones B, Shak S, Fuchs H, Paton V, Bajamonde A, et al. Use of chemotherapy plus a monoclonal antibody against HER2 for metastatic breast cancer that overexpresses HER2. *N Engl J Med* 2001;344:783–92.
- O'Shaughnessy J, Miles D, Vukelja S, Moiseyenko V, Ayoub JP, Cervantes G, et al. Superior survival with capecitabine plus docetaxel combination therapy in anthracycline-pretreated patients with advanced breast cancer: phase III trial results. *J Clin Oncol* 2002;28:12–23.
- Hortobagyi GN, Theriault RL, Porter L, Blaney D, Lipton A, Sinoff C, et al. Efficacy of pamidronate in reducing skeletal complications in patients with breast cancer and lytic bone metastases. *N Engl J Med* 1996;355:1785–91.
- Tannock IF, Boyd NF, DeBoer G, Elrichman C, Fine S, Laroque G, et al. A randomized trial of two dose levels of cyclophosphamide, methotrexate and fluorouracil chemotherapy for patients with metastatic breast cancer. *J Clin Oncol* 1998;6:1377–87.

13 Prognostic factors

AM Thompson, SE Pinder

Prognostic factors are of value for three main reasons:
- To predict outcome for an individual patient
- To allow comparisons of treatment between groups of patients at similar risk of recurrence and death
- To improve our understanding of breast cancer and develop new therapeutic approaches.

Prognostic factors should:
- Have clear biological significance
- Be applicable to clearly defined patient populations
- Be based on robust, reproducible data.

Prognostic factors put individual patients in a low or high risk group that indicates a relative rather than an absolute prediction of the future behaviour of the disease. The patient profile cannot always predict prognosis precisely. The factors often interrelate with each other. Nonetheless, they are useful in guiding therapeutic decisions, and biological factors are becoming more helpful, especially in predicting a patient's response to certain types of treatment.

Clinical factors

Tumour size

The size of a cancer, as measured by the pathologist on the fresh or fixed macroscopic specimen and confirmed or amended after histological examination, correlates with survival. Patients with smaller cancers have a better survival than those with larger tumours.

Axillary status

Axillary nodal metastasis that has been proven by histology is the most powerful prognostic factor in breast cancer in the majority of studies. Survival is correlated directly with the number and level of axillary lymph nodes involved.

Recent interest has focused on the assessment of small deposits of tumour within axillary lymph nodes known as micrometastases. Different definitions for these micrometastases are used with different methods of identification, including step sectioning, immunohistochemistry, and reverse transcription polymerase chain reaction. Their importance, however, is unclear. The new tumour node metastasis staging system uses a pragmatic definition of a micrometastasis as measuring between 0.2 mm and 2 mm in size. Such metastatic foci are categorised as positive nodal disease for staging purposes, with smaller deposits of isolated tumour cells classified as node negative.

Metastatic disease

Patients with metastatic disease, particularly the 10% of patients with metastases at the time of presentation (M1 or stage IV disease), have a poorer prognosis than those with apparently localised disease. Survival differs according to the site of disease. Patients with supraclavicular fossa disease have a better survival than patients with metastatic disease at other sites. Patients with bone metastases and no visceral metastases have a better outlook than those with visceral disease.

Age

Young women (particularly those <35 years) have a poorer prognosis than older women who have the disease at an equivalent stage. Being young is a marker for recurrence of local disease and, hence, distant disease.

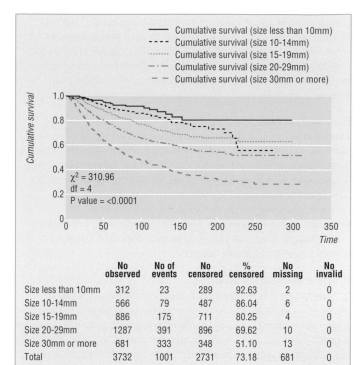

	No observed	No of events	No censored	% censored	No missing	No invalid
Size less than 10mm	312	23	289	92.63	2	0
Size 10-14mm	566	79	487	86.04	6	0
Size 15-19mm	886	175	711	80.25	4	0
Size 20-29mm	1287	391	896	69.62	10	0
Size 30mm or more	681	333	348	51.10	13	0
Total	3732	1001	2731	73.18	681	0

Overall survival by invasive tumour size in 3732 primary operable invasive breast cancers. From Nottingham Tenovus Primary Breast Cancer Series

Survival of patients with breast cancer according to involvement of axillary lymph nodes

Lymph node involvement	Survival at 10 years (%)
All patients	66
Negative axillary nodes	77
Positive axillary nodes	45
1–3	51
≥4	30

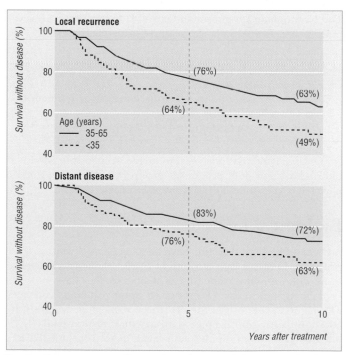

Freedom from recurrence of cancer in patients in relation to age when breast cancer first diagnosed. (Proportional hazards model showed women <35 to have relative risk of 1.6 for distant disease)

Histological factors

Histological grade

Histological grade is assessed on tubule formation, nuclear pleomorphism, and mitotic frequency, and the assessment is done by a trained pathologist. Three histological grades (1, 2, and 3) correlate with survival. The quality of fixation (and hence preservation of cellular architecture) is critical in determining the tumour grade accurately.

Histological type

Special types of invasive breast cancer, including tubular, mucinous, and invasive cribriform cancer, are associated with a better prognosis than invasive ductal cancer of no special type. In addition, histological type provides information about the biological behaviour of invasive breast carcinoma—for example, invasive lobular carcinomas will probably be oestrogen receptor positive, lack p53 expression, have a low proliferation rate, and metastasise in a different pattern of spread to invasive ductal cancers.

Lymphovascular invasion

In the breast, it is not possible to distinguish histologically lymphatic channels from blood vessels on routine haematoxylin and eosin stained sections, so the term lymphovascular invasion is used. Tumour cells in the lumen of lymphovascular channels are present in up to a quarter of patients with breast cancer. Lymphovascular invasion is associated with local disease recurrence and a high risk of short term systemic relapse.

Other histological markers

Peritumoral angiogenesis and micrometastases within draining lymph nodes (whether detected by histology, immunohistochemistry, or molecular enrichment techniques such as the polymerase chain reaction) require more evidence to determine if they have any prognostic importance.

Prognostic indices

Many histological and biological factors that determine prognosis are interrelated. Some are difficult to determine, and many do not have confirmed independent prognostic value. The Nottingham prognostic index (NPI) incorporates invasive tumour size, lymph node status, and histological grade.

> **Nottingham Prognostic Index =**
> **0.2 × invasive size in cm**
> **+ lymph node stage (score 1 for no nodes, 2 for 1–3 nodes, 3 for ≥ 4 nodes)**
> **+ grade (score 1 for grade 1, 2 for grade 2, 3 for grade 3)**

Originally the NPI was used to divide women into good, intermediate, or poor prognostic groups. Confirmatory studies have led to a refined NPI with five categories.

Biological factors

A range of biological factors have been associated with prognosis in breast cancer, often in small, selected series and some without multivariate statistical analysis. Few have confirmed clinical use. Oestrogen receptor protein is associated with a good prognosis in the first three years after diagnosis. In addition, oestrogen receptor status predicts response to hormone treatment. Epidermal growth factor receptor (HER1) correlates inversely with oestrogen receptor and is associated with reduced survival. HER2 (formerly CerbB2/neu) is associated with poor prognosis in node positive patients.

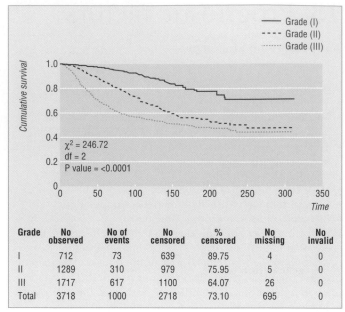

Grade	No observed	No of events	No censored	% censored	No missing	No invalid
I	712	73	639	89.75	4	0
II	1289	310	979	75.95	5	0
III	1717	617	1100	64.07	26	0
Total	3718	1000	2718	73.10	695	0

Overall survival by histological grade in 3718 primary operable invasive breast cancers. Adapted from Nottingham Tenovus Primary Breast Cancer Series

Nottingham prognostic index

Group	Index value	Survival at 10 years (%)
Excellent (EPG)	2.0–2.4	96
Good (GPG)	2.41–3.4	93
Moderate 1 (MPG 1)	3.41–4.4	82
Moderate 2 (MPG 2)	4.41–5.4	75
Poor (PPG)	5.41–6.4	53
Very poor (VPPG)	≥ 6.41	39

There has been a dramatic improvement in survival over the last decade as shown in significantly improved data from the Nottingham Tenovus Primary Breast Cancer Series. These data relate to patients with primary operable breast cancer treated from 1990 to 1996

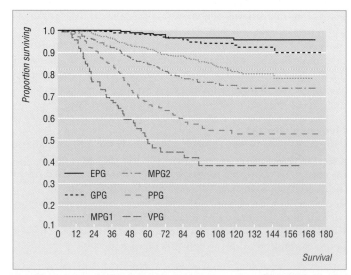

Overall survival by Nottingham prognostic index group (1990–96 data). EPG = excellent prognostic group, GPG = good prognostic group, MPG1 = moderate 1 prognostic group, MPG2 = moderate 2 prognostic group, PPG = poor prognostic group, VPG = very poor prognostic group. From Nottingham Tenovus Primary Breast Cancer Series

These three markers have different therapeutic approaches.
- Oestrogen receptor—tamoxifen, selective oestrogen receptor modulators, and aromatase inhibitors
- Epidermal growth factor receptor— gefitinib (currently in clinical trials)
- HER2—trastuzumab (herceptin)

Many other biological markers are of uncertain clinical significance.

Biological markers of uncertain clinical significance

- Proliferation markers—Ki67*, MIB1*, thymidine labelling, %S phase, topoisomerase II alpha, mitotic activity index
- Apoptosis regulating genes—bcl2*, bcl-x, bax, bak, survivin
- Cell cycle regulatory genes—cyclin A, B, D*, E; overexpression of p21*, p27, p53*
- Cell adhesion molecules—E cadherin*, integrins, fibronectin, MSF
- Proteases—cathepsin D, matrix metalloproteinase, tissue inhibitor of matrix metalloproteinases
- Oncogenes—HER3, HER4
- Oestrogen receptor related—progesterone receptor*, pS2
- Signal transduction pathways—extracellular signal regulated kinase 1/2, J N-terminal kinase, and p38
- Allelic imbalance—1p, 7q, 8p, 10q, 11q, 15q, 17p*, 17q*

---

* Denotes biological markers for which a number of studies have shown an association with outcome

Future

Tissue microarrays, in which 0.6 mm cores from histology paraffin blocks of many samples are aligned next to each other on a single slide, allow the evaluation of a large number of cases on a single histological section. They have been used in the evaluation of marker expression by immunohistochemistry in breast cancer. In addition, RNA and DNA based microarray technology, which examines thousands of genes on a single slide, has been used to assess the relation between gene expression and outcome in several series. A range of complex statistical techniques show that clusters of some 70 genes (including some of those mentioned above) have been associated putatively with prognosis in breast cancer, and there has been confirmation of their clinical value. Proteomic arrays to examine expression of known and novel proteins in tissues or serum from patients present alternative markers of response to therapy and may be related to prognosis.

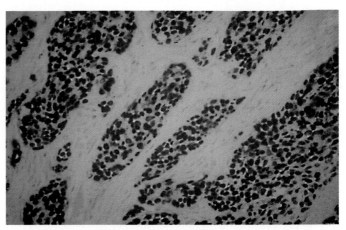

Oestrogen receptor alpha stained breast cancer

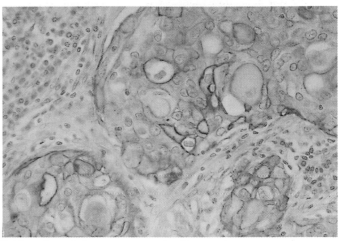

Epidermal growth factor receptor stained breast cancer

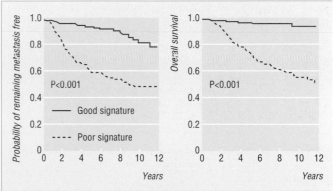

Patient outcome based on genetic profile of primary tumour. Patients classified on basis of 78 genes as having good signatures or poor signature. The 70 genes included those involved in invasion, metastases, angiogenesis, and signal transduction. Adapted from van de Vijver MJ et al. *N Engl J Med* 2002;347:1999–2009

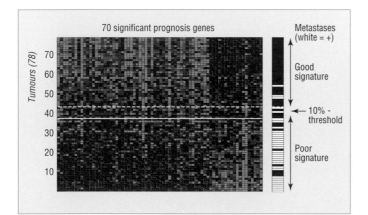

Microarray results from 70 significant genes in the Amsterdam study. These genes identify cancers with good or poor prognostic signatures. The genes came from 78 patients who were aged under 55 with breast cancers that were lymph node negative. These patients had no adjuvant therapy and 34 developed distant metastases within five years and 44 had no distant metastases within five years

> Although many prognostic molecular markers with a range of techniques are under evaluation, established clinical and pathological markers are the prognostic features of clinical relevance

Certain internet sites provide useful information on individual patient prognosis and give an outline of likely benefits from different adjuvant therapies.

www.adjuvantonline.com is a constantly updated site that provides information on the probability of relapse and survival using patient details including age, general health, oestrogen receptor status, tumour size, grade, and node status. It provides details of recurrence rates and survival with and without adjuvant therapy and the likely benefits in terms of reduction of recurrence and improvements in survival from different endocrine and chemotherapy adjuvant therapies.

Further reading

- Veronesi U, Galimberti V, Zurrida S, Merson M, Greco M, Luini A. Prognostic significance of number and level of axillary node metastases in breast cancer. *Breast* 1993;3:224–8.
- Singletary SA, Allred C, Ashley P, Bassett LW, Berry D, Bland KI, et al. Revision of the American Joint Committee on cancer staging system for breast cancer staging. *J Clin Oncol* 2002;20:3628–36.
- Vrieling C, Collette L, Fourquet A, Hoogenraad WJ, Horiot J-C, Jager J, et al. Can patient-, treatment- and pathology-related characteristics explain the high local recurrence rate following breast-conserving therapy in young patients? *Eur J Cancer* 2003;39:932–44.
- Elston CW, Ellis IO. Pathological prognostic factors in breast cancer. I. The value of histological grade in breast cancer: experience from a large study with long-term follow-up. *Histopathology* 1991;19:403–10.
- Galea MH, Blamey RW, Elston CE, Ellis IO. The Nottingham Prognostic Index in primary breast cancer. *Breast Cancer Res Treat* 1992;22:207–19.
- Van de Vijver MJ, Yudong DH, Van t'Veer LJ, Dai H, Hart AA, Voskuil DW, et al. A gene expression signature as a predictor of survival in breast cancer. *N Engl J Med* 2002;34:1999–2009.
- Van't Veer L, Dai H, Van de Vijver MJ, Yudong DH, Augustinus A, Hart M, et al. Ge expression profiling predicts clinical outcome of breast cancer. *Nature* 2002;415:530–36.

The sources of the data presented in the graphs are: Nixon AJ et al. *J Clin Oncol* 1994;12:888–94 for disease free survival related to age, the Nottingham Tenovus Primary Operable Breast Cancer Series for graphs comparing tumour size, histological grade and Nottingham prognostic index group to survival. The immunohistochemical sections are courtesy of SE Pinder (oestrogen receptor alpha), SE Pinder (epidermal growth factor receptor)

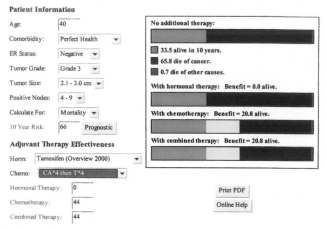

Print outs from adjuvantonline.com showing calculations for relapse and potential benefits of treatment with five years aromatase inhibitors and anthracyclines in a postmenopausal patient with oestrogen receptor positive breast cancer (top) and calculation for mortality for a second younger (premenopausal) patient with oestrogen receptor negative high risk disease treated with a combination of an anthracycline and a taxane (bottom)

14 Clinical trials of management of early breast cancer

JR Yarnold

Importance of clinical trials

New treatments are evaluated in well defined stages. Phase I trials identify dose limiting toxicities and safe dose schedules. Phase II studies test for a predefined rate of tumour response in selected cohorts of patients. Phase III trials test the balance of beneficial and adverse clinical effects and cost effectiveness in patients representative of the target population. If a new treatment is much better than previous treatments, as was the case when antibiotics were first introduced, clinical evaluation is easy.

Cancer treatment is not like that. It requires rigorous testing to detect modest clinical benefits. Comparisons are vulnerable to systematic and random errors unless randomisation and adequate sample size are incorporated into trial design. Systematic errors are introduced if the method of allocating patients to one or other treatment is biased in terms of factors (for example, stage of tumour, age of patient, other treatment undertaken) known to influence outcome. To eliminate bias, treatment allocation is determined by randomisation, a key feature of phase III clinical trials. Randomisation cannot secure a perfect balance of all known (and unknown) factors that influence outcome because chance introduces imbalances (in the same way that a coin tossed 10 times does not always land on five heads and five tails). The more patients who are randomised, however, the smaller these random imbalances are, and the greater the chance that differences in outcome can be attributed reliably to the randomised intervention, usually a treatment.

Large multicentre trials are necessary to show that modest survival differences between trial arms are not caused by random imbalances in prognostic factors. In practice, several thousand patients are needed to reliably attribute a 5% improvement in survival to treatment rather than to chance. Data from different trials can be combined for meta-analysis to increase confidence that small treatment effects are reliably detected. Better still, systematic overviews collect data on every patient in every randomised trial undertaken. This has been the outstanding achievement of the Early Breast Cancer Trialists' Collaborative Group (EBCTCG), whose analyses are discussed in this chapter. Most clinical trials have evaluated four different forms of treatment for women in operable breast cancer—surgery, radiotherapy, endocrine therapy, and chemotherapy.

Surgery

Early trials compared radical mastectomy (removal of breast, axillary lymph nodes, and pectoral muscles) with supraradical procedures (removing the above plus supraclavicular, internal mammary, and mediastinal nodes) as a test of the original Halsted hypothesis of contiguous tumour spread. No survival advantage was seen after more extensive surgery. Trials to evaluate less radical alternatives to mastectomy were started in the 1970s. A landmark study from Milan compared radical mastectomy with quadrantectomy (removal of the quadrant of the breast in which the tumour was situated) plus radiotherapy to the breast. No statistically significant differences in disease free and overall survival were detected. Since then, a systematic overview of all relevant surgical trials has confirmed the

Categories of treatments for early breast cancer investigated by clinical trials

- Extent of primary surgery
- Postoperative radiotherapy
- Endocrine therapy
- Chemotherapy

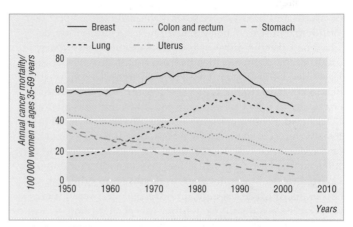

Trends since 1950 in age standardised (35–69 years) death rates comparing breast and selected other types of cancer among women in the United Kingdom. The fall in mortality since 1990 has been mainly caused by the introduction of adjuvant therapy as a consequence of results from clinical trials

For a disease as common as breast cancer, an improvement in survival of 5% at 10 years translates into many hundreds of thousands of deaths prevented worldwide

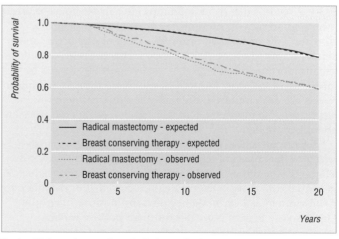

Kaplan-Meier estimate of survival after radical mastectomy or breast conserving therapy (quandrantectomy, axillary dissection, and radiotherapy). The lower curves correspond to observed survival, taking into account deaths from any cause. The upper curves (almost identical) show the expected survival rate on the basis of mortality ranges in cohorts of Italian women who were age matched

equivalence of mastectomy and breast preserving surgery plus radiotherapy in terms of disease free and overall survival.

For decades, breast cancer specialists debated the influence of local cancer recurrence on the risk of first metastasis and premature death. The National Surgical Adjuvant Breast and Bowel Project B06 (NSABP B06) trial was established to test the importance of local control in the breast on outcome. The B06 trial analysed 1851 women with early breast cancer randomised to simple mastectomy, tumour excision (lumpectomy), or tumour excision plus breast radiotherapy, with all women having axillary dissection. Overall survival at 20 years was not significantly different between any of the arms of the trial. However, a threefold reduction in local recurrence risk after tumour excision plus radiotherapy (78 local recurrences) compared with tumour excision alone (220 local recurrences) was associated with a statistically significant reduction in metastasis and breast cancer death (hazard ratio 0.82; 95% confidence interval 0.68 to 0.99). The association must be causal because the only way that local treatments (surgery, radiotherapy) influence deaths from breast cancer is by the prevention of first metastasis. This important trial showed that local recurrence in the breast is the source of first metastasis in a minority (5–10%) of women treated by lumpectomy alone. Level I evidence from a series of trials conducted in Milan showed that surgical margins are important determinants of local recurrence risk after breast conservation surgery. In the B06 trial, the benefit of better local control after radiotherapy is partially offset by an increase in deaths from other causes. This explains why no significant difference in overall survival was seen. Excess deaths from other causes may relate to adverse effects of radiotherapy on the heart in patients with left sided tumours.

Radiotherapy

The systematic overview by the EBCTCG of 17 000 women entered in trials testing radiotherapy confirms that postmastectomy radiotherapy to the chest wall reduces the annual odds of local recurrence by 68% (SE 2.3). In women treated in the 1960s and 1970s, chest wall radiotherapy prevented ≥20 local recurrences at 10 years for every 100 women treated. The same magnitude of benefit was seen in the NSABP B06 trial of radiotherapy after breast conserving surgery. According to the systematic overview, the prevention of 20 local recurrences by radiotherapy after mastectomy or breast conservation surgery prevents five breast cancer deaths at 10 years. This remarkably favourable ratio of one breast cancer death prevented for every four local recurrences prevented has been undermined in the past by excess mortality caused by cardiovascular disease induced by radiation. If heart and major vessels are excluded from the radiotherapy treatment volume, it is reasonable to assume that this cause of iatrogenic mortality no longer applies.

A more intriguing question probed by radiotherapy trials relates to the impact of regional lymphatic (especially axillary) relapse on overall survival. In a systematic overview, the reduction in annual risk of breast cancer death reported after radiotherapy is the same in axillary node negative and positive subgroups. The absolute benefit is greater for node positive women, representing up to 10 fewer deaths from breast cancer at 10 years per 100 node positive women irradiated. The inference is that control of axillary disease prevents first metastasis and premature death in an important minority of women. This inference holds regardless of how regional control is achieved (by radiotherapy, surgery, or systemic therapy).

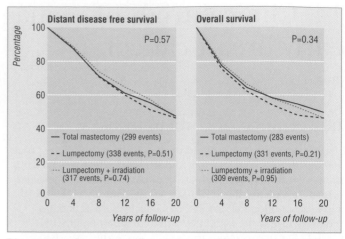

Distant disease free and overall survival among 589 women treated with total mastectomy, 634 treated with lumpectomy alone and 628 treated with lumpectomy plus radiotherapy

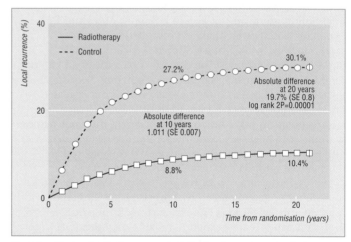

Absolute affects of radiotherapy on isolated local recurrence as first event

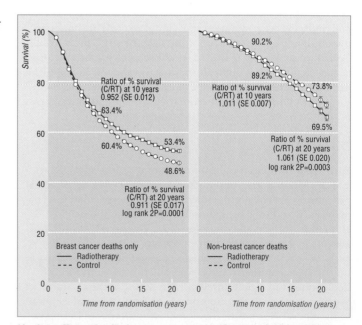

Absolute effects of radiotherapy on cause-specific survival. (C = control, RT = radiotherapy)

Endocrine therapy

Ovarian ablation

Trials started before 1980 testing ovarian ablation by surgery or radiotherapy in >2000 women confirmed a substantial overall survival benefit for women <50 years randomised to ovarian ablation. As the benefit shows no signs of diminishing 15 years after randomisation, it is conceivable that this represents permanent cure of a few patients rather than postponement of metastasis and death. Women allocated ovarian suppression in the absence of chemotherapy gain a 24% (SD 7) reduction in the annual odds of death, amounting to an absolute benefit of 5.6% in axillary node negative women and 12.5% in node positive women. Retrospective subgroup analysis confirms that the benefit is confined to the oestrogen receptor positive subgroup, representing roughly 75% of tumours. These benefits are not seen in the presence of chemotherapy, presumably because of ovarian failure induced by cytotoxic drugs in older premenopausal women. Since these early trials were conducted, the effectiveness of luteinising hormone releasing hormone agonists has been confirmed as an alternative to surgical or radiotherapeutic ablation. Issues being dealt with in trials yet to report include the added benefits of cytotoxic therapy in addition to ovarian ablation, and the benefits of tamoxifen or aromatase inhibitors against a background of ovarian ablation in premenopausal women.

Tamoxifen

Randomised trials involving 30 000 women confirm that five years of tamoxifen in women with oestrogen receptor positive disease reduces the annual odds of death by 31% (SE 3), corresponding to an absolute overall survival benefit at 10 years of 10.9% in node positive patients and 5.6% in node negative patients. Women <50 years gain the same benefits as older women as long as they take the drug for five years. Trials testing tamoxifen against a background of chemotherapy (chemotherapy versus chemotherapy and tamoxifen) confirm that tamoxifen effects are independent of cytotoxic treatment (unlike ovarian ablation). Small trials of several hundred women have tested the importance of sequencing of cytotoxic drugs and tamoxifen. They have reported a small but statistically significant disadvantage in terms of disease free survival with concurrent tamoxifen and chemotherapy compared to tamoxifen introduced after chemotherapy. Other questions being investigated by clinical trials include the benefits (or otherwise) of continuing tamoxifen beyond five years.

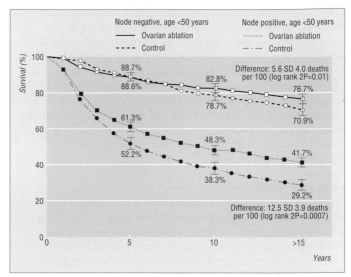

Absolute effects of ovarian ablation in the absence of chemotherapy on overall survival among women under 50 years at entry

> Adjuvant tamoxifen for five years reduces annual breast cancer death rate by 31% (SE 3) irrespective of the use of chemotherapy and of age. For oestrogen receptor positive tumours the annual breast cancer mortality rates are similar during years 0–4 and 5–15. Five years of tamoxifen produces the same proportional reductions over 15 years, so that cumulative reduction in mortality is more than twice as large at 15 years as it is at five years

Effects of tamoxifen for about five years according to oestrogen receptor level oestrogen receptor level

Oestrogen receptor level	Reduction (SE) in annual odds		
	Recurrence	Breast cancer death	Any death
Poor (<10 fmol/mg)	−4 (7%)	−4 (8%)	−3 (7%)
Positive (≥10, <100 fmol/mg)	36 (4%)	27 (5%)	22 (5%)
Positive (≥100 fmol/mg)	49 (5%)	45 (6%)	33 (5%)
Unknown	31 (7%)	20 (9%)	14 (8%)

Unanticipated outcomes of the early adjuvant tamoxifen trials, since confirmed by systematic overview, include a reduction in the annual risk of contralateral breast cancer. This

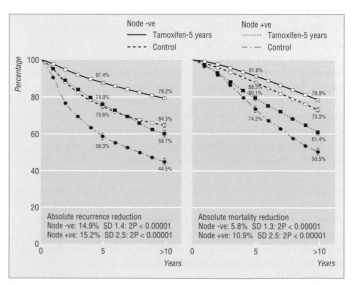

Absolute risk reductions for recurrence and survival during the first 10 years, subdivided by tamoxifen duration and by nodal status (after exclusion of women with oestrogen receptor poor disease)

ranges from 13% (SD 13) for trials of one year of tamoxifen to 25% (SD 9) for two years of tamoxifen and 49% (SD 9) for five years of the drug. Current trials testing adjuvant aromatase inhibitors against tamoxifen include the incidence of contralateral primary breast cancers as secondary endpoints, with early indications that aromatase inhibitors achieve further reductions in risk than those achieved by tamoxifen. The overview also confirms a doubling of the risk of endometrial cancer in patients who receive tamoxifen treatment for two years, corresponding to one additional case per several thousand women per year.

Aromatase inhibitors

The clinical benefits of complete oestrogen blockade in postmenopausal women are seen in the effects of aromatase inhibitors, drugs that reduce postmenopausal circulating oestrogen levels to the lower limits of detection. Data from the first trial that compared adjuvant tamoxifen and anastrazole in >9000 women confirm better disease free survival in women randomised to anastrazole, but no overall survival is evident as yet. Other trials have shown the benefit of letrozole as first line treatment, and patients who switched to exemestane or anastrozole after two or three years of tamoxifen also had a significant reduction in breast cancer events. Further evidence consistent with the effectiveness of these drugs comes from a trial that randomised women after five years tamoxifen between the aromatase inhibitor letrozole and placebo. Application of preagreed stopping rules caused the premature termination of the trial (median follow-up 2.4 years) with the emergence of an early disease free survival gain with letrozole, which led to the offer of letrozole to all women in the placebo group. A subsequent analysis showed a survival benefit on patients who were node positive at diagnosis.

Chemotherapy

The EBCTCG systematic overview evaluated 17 000 women randomised into 47 trials that compared several months of polychemotherapy (most commonly cyclophosphamide, methotrexate, 5 fluorouracil, (CMF)) with no chemotherapy. These trials conducted between 1973 and 1989 confirm a 27% (SD 5) reduction in annual risk of death for up to 10 years in women younger than 50 and a 11% (SD 3) reduction for women aged 50–69. Only a few hundred women over the age of 70 have been entered into trials, so little can be said about this important age group. The large number of women in these trials supports retrospective subgroup analyses of a range of factors that influence outcome. For example, the relative benefit (reduction in the annual odds/risk of death) falls with patient age, but it is independent of tumour stage. The absolute benefits (number of deaths prevented per 100 women treated) depend on age and prognosis, and they are greatest for young women with node positive cancer. Subgroup analyses confirm that women with oestrogen receptor positive and oestrogen receptor negative tumours benefit from chemotherapy, with a suggestion of greater benefit if the tumour is oestrogen receptor negative. The therapeutic benefits of chemotherapy seem the same whether tamoxifen is given or not, an important observation consistent with independent and additive effects. Tamoxifen should, however, be given after chemotherapy has finished. Review of a subgroup of almost 7000 women randomised to anthracycline-containing regimens versus CMF in 11 trials between 1973 and 1989 lends strong support to the superiority of regimens containing anthracycline. The absolute benefit depends on prognosis and age, ranging from one to several

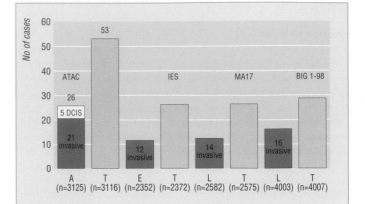

Incidence of new contralateral breast primaries in ongoing adjuvant aromatase inhibitor adjuvant trials. A = anastrozole, ATAC = arimidex or tamoxifen alone or in combination, BIG 1–98 = Breast International Group, E = exemestane, IES = intergroup exemestane study, MA17 = study coordinated by the Canadian Breast Cancer Group, T = tamoxifen

Six months of anthracycline based polychemotherapy reduces the annual breast cancer death rate by about 38% (SE 5) for women <50 years, and about 25% (SE 4) for those women who are 50–69 years, irrespective of the use of tamoxifen and oestrogen receptor status. Anthracycline regimens are significantly more effective than CMF chemotherapy

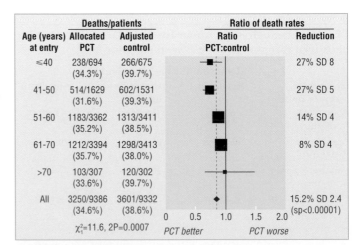

Proportional risk reductions in death from any cause with polychemotherapy, subdivided by age at randomisation. (PCT = polychemotherapy)

fewer deaths at 10 years for every 100 women treated with anthracylines compared with those treated with CMF.

Several randomised clinical trials involving a few thousand women have tested the effects of neoadjuvant (before surgery) versus adjuvant (after surgery) chemotherapy in women with early breast cancer. No mortality differences were reported. In patients who would otherwise need mastectomy (for example, for a large tumour), neoadjuvant chemotherapy improves the chances of breast conservation surgery. Although no systematic overview of high dose chemotherapy has been undertaken, a series of trials has detected no significant clinical benefit in terms of mortality in any defined subgroups. Trials involving many thousands of patients have tested the benefits of adjuvant schedules containing a taxane (paclitaxel or docetaxel) compared with a non-taxane standard. Conflicting results from different trials have failed to clarify the value of adding taxanes as adjuvant therapy. One study comparing anthracyclines with or without added taxane did show a survival advantage for the combination.

> For middle aged women with oestrogen receptor positive disease, the breast cancer mortality rate over 15 years is about halved by six months of anthracycline based chemotherapy followed by five years of adjuvant tamoxifen

Estimated effects of six months of chemotherapy based on anthracycline or five years of tamoxifen, or both, on 15 year breast cancer mortality (%), in the absence of other causes of death*

Systemic adjuvant treatment and age at diagnosis (years)	Proportional effect on annual breast cancer mortality rate treatment v control)		15 year breast cancer mortality with treatment (risk (%) and absolute gain) v corresponding risk without treatment					
	Ratio of rates	Proportional reduction	Low risk (for example, small tumour node negative		Moderate risk (for example, large tumour node negative)		High risk (for example, any tumour size node positive)	
			Risk	Gain	Risk	Gain	Risk	Gain
Chemotherapy only in oestrogen receptor poor or oestrogen receptor positive disease†								
None (any age)	1.0		12.5		25.0		50.0	
Anthracycline¶ (age<50 years)	0.62	38%	7.9	4.6	16.3	8.7	34.9	15.1
Anthracycline¶ (50–69 years)‡	0.80	205	10.1	2.4	20.6	4.4	42.6	7.4
Endocrine or chemoendocrine therapy in oestrogen receptor positive disease†								
None (any age)	1.0		12.5		25.0		50.0	
Tamoxifen§(any age)	0.60	31%	8.8	3.7	18.0	7.0	38.0	12.0
Anthracycline¶ plus tamoxifen§ (age<50 years)	0.62 × 0.69	57%	5.6	6.9	11.6	13.4	25.7	24.3
Anthracycline¶ plus tamoxifen§ (50–69 years)‡	0.80 × 0.69	45%	7.1	5.4	14.7	10.3	31.8	18.2

*Relevance of ER status, age, and underlying risk (10–15%, 25%, or 50%)

†For women of given nodal status the five year mortality is greater for oestrogen receptor poor than oestrogen receptor positive, but the 15 year risks may be similar

‡No reliable data in women older than 69 years

§About five years of adjuvant tamoxifen

¶Anthracycline: about six months of anthracycline-based adjuvant chemotherapy with regimens such as fluorouracil, doxorubicin, and cyclophosphamide or fluorouracil, epirubicin, and cyclophosphamide

Future

The future of phase III clinical trials in breast cancer needs greater national and international collaboration to speed up the evaluation process and complete the accrual of several thousand patients in months rather than years. A potential problem is that outcome requires several years of follow up before conclusions can be drawn from enough deaths. For this reason, disease free survival is increasingly being used as the primary endpoint of effect because these events occur several years before death. Whether disease free survival is a reliable surrogate remains to be seen.

Further reading

- Early Breast Cancer Trialists' Collaborative Group. Favourable and unfavourable effects on long-term survival of radiotherapy for early breast cancer: an overview of the randomised trials. *Lancet* 2000;355:1757–70.
- Early Breast Cancer Trialists' Collaborative Group. Ovarian ablation in early breast cancer: overview of the randomised trials. *Lancet* 1996;348:1189–96.
- Early Breast Cancer Trialists' Collaborative Group. Tamoxifen for early breast cancer: an overview of the randomised trials. *Lancet* 1998;351:1451–67.
- Early Breast Cancer Trialists' Collaborative Group. Effects of chemotherapy and hormonal therapy for early breast cancer on recurrence and 15-year survival: an overview of the randomised trials. *Lancet* 2005;365:1687–1717.

International collaboration is also stimulated by the need to test drugs that target cancers in specific subgroups of patients—for example, the 20% of patients whose tumours overexpress cerbB2 protein as a result of gene amplification benefit from the addition of the adjuvant trastuzumab for one or two years. This points the way to a future of testing drugs that target specific molecular pathways deregulated by cancer gene mutations in different tumour types. It is also possible that initial evaluation of these newer biological drugs would be accelerated by the increased use of the primary tumour as an experimental system rather than occult metastases. This has been an active research field for over a decade, and evaluating tumour changes after short term courses of drugs given before an operation or as neoadjuvant treatment will probably increase in future.

The sources of the data presented in illustrations are: Veronesi U et al. *N Engl J Med* 2002;347:1227–32 for the graph of survival after quadrantectomy or radical mastectomy; Fisher B et al. *N Engl J Med* 2002;347:1233–41 for the graph of survival after wide local excision +/− radiotherapy versus total mastectomy; Early Breast Cancer Trialists' Collaborative Group (EBCTCG), *Lancet* 2000;355:1757–70 for the graphs showing the reductions in breast cancer deaths and excess non-breast cancer deaths in women randomised to radiotherapy after primary surgery; EBCTCG, *Lancet* 1996;348;1189–96 for the graph of effects of ovarian ablation on mortality in the absence of chemotherapy; EBCTCG, *Lancet* 1998;351:1451–67 for the graphs of effects of tamoxifen on mortality in node negative and positive women; in the absence of chemotherapy on survival; EBCTCG, *Lancet* 1998;352:930–42 for the graph of absolute survival advantages during polychemotherapy. The data are reproduced with permission of the journals or copyright holders. The final table is modified from *Lancet* 2005;365:1687–717.

15 Psychological aspects

P Maguire, P Hopwood

Psychological morbidity

Most women who present with breast lumps are emotionally distressed. A substantial proportion of women whose lumps prove to be benign remain distressed, however, and they may become clinically anxious or depressed, particularly if they have chronic breast pain.

Up to 30% of women with breast cancer develop an anxiety state or depressive illness within a year of diagnosis, which is three to four times the expected rate in matched community samples. After mastectomy, 20–30% of patients develop persisting problems with body image and sexual difficulties. Breast conserving surgery reduces problems with body image, but this may be offset by increased fears of recurrence. Consequently, less surgery does not mean less psychiatric morbidity. Immediate breast reconstruction after mastectomy may reduce this morbidity, provided that the possible complications have been discussed fully and understood, that the patient wants it for herself and not because of pressure from others, and that it is carried out expertly. Psychiatric morbidity further increases when radiotherapy or chemotherapy is used.

Problems of recognition

Few patients mention psychological morbidity because they do not think that it is acceptable to do so. Doctors can promote disclosure of such problems by asking questions and clarifying the responses about patients' perceptions of the nature of their illness, their reactions to it, and about their experience of losing a breast or having radiotherapy or chemotherapy. By being empathic, making educated guesses about how a patient is feeling, and summarising what has been disclosed, doctors promote disclosure and expression of related feelings.

Disclosure is inhibited by closed, leading, and multiple questions and by giving advice and reassurance, especially if important problems have not been disclosed. If the questions asked in the first few minutes of a consultation focus on physical aspects only, patients will assume that they should not discuss other problems. If problems are not disclosed despite encouragement, it is useful to ask about the impact of the illness on several key areas: daily functioning since surgery, relationship with a partner, and mood.

When there is any hint of anxiety or depression, clinicians should inquire about key symptoms by asking open directive questions ("What changes have you noticed while you have been depressed? How have you been sleeping?"). Patients with problems with their body image should be asked how much they avoid looking at their chest wall and how they react if they catch sight of it. In patients with sexual difficulties, doctors should check whether they represent a new problem and explore the reactions of patients and their partners.

Treatment

Anxiety and depression

Patients who have a core mood change but too few symptoms to justify a clinical diagnosis usually respond to understanding and emotional support and do not merit psychiatric referral, especially given the stigma associated with such a referral. The treatment of an anxiety state depends on its severity. A patient who is struggling to cope should be given a benzodiazepine

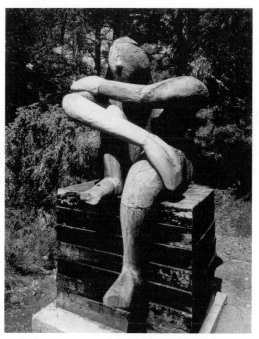

Sculpture of a woman who has had a mastectomy and who is curled up and withdrawn (by Elspeth Bennie)

Reasons for non-disclosure of psychological morbidity
- Problems are inevitable
- Problems cannot be alleviated
- To avoid burdening health professionals
- To avoid being judged inadequate
- Relevant questions not asked by health professionals
- Cues met by distancing, such as "you are bound to be upset"

Disclosure by patients

Inhibited by	Promoted by
• Closed questions	• Open directive question
• Leading questions	• Questions with a psychological focus
• Multiple questions	• Clarification of psychological aspects
• Questions with a physical focus	• Summarising
• Offering advice or reassurance especially if premature	• Screening questions
	• Empathy
	• Educated guesses

Criteria for an anxiety state
- Persistent anxiety, tension, or inability to relax
- Present for more than half of the time for four weeks
- Cannot pull self out of it or be distracted by others
- Substantial departure from normal mood

Plus at least four of the following:
- Initial insomnia
- Irritability
- Impaired concentration
- Intolerance of noise
- Panic attacks
- Somatic manifestation

(for example, diazepam) to be used as needed for up to three weeks—this avoids the risk of dependency—or a small dose of an antipsychotic drug (for example, chlorpromazine 25 mg three times a day). Once a patient reports some improvement, it is worth teaching them techniques for managing anxiety. This is helpful as further anxiety is often triggered by mention of breast cancer in the media, new physical symptoms, or attendance at clinic. When somatic symptoms of anxiety predominate, the use of a β blocker (for example, propranolol) should be considered.

Depressive illness responds well to antidepressant drugs given in therapeutic doses for four to six months. Doctors should explain that the drugs, unlike tranquillisers, do not cause physical dependence—they reverse the biochemical changes caused by the shock of diagnosis and treatment. Stressing that any other problems will be dealt with once the mood has begun to improve also improves compliance. Agitated patients benefit from a sedating drug (for example, dothiepin, initially 75 mg at night increasing to up to 150 mg). Patients who are apathetic and lethargic benefit from an alerting agent (for example, fluoxetine 20 mg in the morning). If anxiety, depression, or any underlying problems persist, psychiatric referral should be considered especially if there is any hint of suicide.

Conditioned responses

Up to a quarter of patients who receive combination chemotherapy develop conditioned responses. Any stimulus that reminds them of treatment causes them to reflexively experience adverse effects such as nausea and vomiting. Phobic reactions can develop, which make further chemotherapy difficult. Although new antiemetics, such as ondansetron, have reduced this problem, conditioned responses need to be recognised and treated promptly. Covering each infusion with an anxiolytic drug (for example, lorazepam 2 mg three times a day as needed) for 48 hours before and during treatment is often effective.

Body image and sexual problems

When surgical reconstruction is possible, patients must have a chance to talk at length about possible complications as well as advantages and to look at photographs of a range of outcomes. Patients who are ineligible for or who refuse surgery may benefit from graded exposure to views of the chest wall of patients after various procedures or cognitive therapy carried out by a clinical psychologist. Sexual difficulties usually require the attention of a sex therapist.

Prevention

Breaking bad news

The first step is to check a patient's idea about what is wrong. This will often be that the lump is cancerous. The doctor should confirm that this is correct, pause to let this sink in, acknowledge the patient's distress, and establish what concerns are contributing to this distress. Only then should reassurance, information, and advice be offered. Before doing so, the doctor can ask if the patient has brought someone with her and if she would like this person to be present while her concerns are discussed. Provision of tape recordings of the consultation may also facilitate psychological adaptation.

If a patient does not know she has cancer, the doctor might say, "The lump is more serious than we thought", and then pause to allow a response such as, "I'll leave the details to you, you're the expert", or, "What do you mean, serious?" The latter type of response indicates a wish to know more, and the doctor should then offer a further euphemism: "The biopsy found some abnormal cells". The patient can pull out of the dialogue

Criteria for depressive illness

- Persistent low mood
- Present for more than half of the time for four weeks
- Cannot be distracted out of it by self or others
- Qualitatively or quantitatively significantly different from normal mood
- Inability to enjoy oneself
- Plus at least four of the following:
  — Diurnal variation of mood
  — Repeated or early waking
  — Impaired concentration or indecisiveness
  — Feeling hopeless or suicidal
  — Feelings of guilt, self blame, being a burden, or worthlessness
  — Irritability and anger for no reason
  — Loss of interest
  — Retardation or agitation

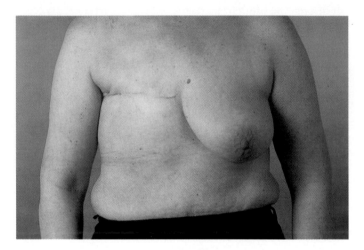

Mastectomy can lead to problems with body images

Preventing psychological morbidity

- Elicit patient's awareness of diagnosis
- If patient is unaware "test water" by using euphemisms and tailor statements according to patient's responses
- If patient is aware, confirm diagnosis:
  — Pause to let news sink in
  — Acknowledge subsequent distress
  — Establish contributive concerns
  — Check patient's needs for information
  — Give information and advice
  — When appropriate discuss treatment options

> When a patient is unaware that she has cancer, the doctor should give a "warning shot" to check if the patient wants to pull out of or move on to the process of truth telling

or ask for further details. The doctor can then say, "I'm afraid it's cancer", and, after pausing, proceed as described above. This way of breaking bad news reduces the risk of provoking denial or overwhelming distress.

Denial

Some patients will not respond to the warnings about the seriousness of their condition. Even so, they will usually ask about treatment. If not, they should be asked whether they would like to know what can be done. When patients reject the need for treatment, their denial should be challenged, as described in the management of recurrence.

Relatives' views

Relatives may insist that a patient should not be told. They may want to protect her from anguish or believe that she would not cope with the bad news. Their reasons should be explored but respected. They should be invited to reflect on the potential costs to them personally and to their relationship and then asked if they would allow the patient's perception of her condition to be explored. If the patient thinks that she has breast cancer, the doctor should confirm that she is correct and proceed as after breaking bad news. If she is not aware of her condition, she should be left in denial.

Preference for treatment

It is important to check if a patient has a strong preference for a particular treatment and to honour this when it is technically possible or to explain why it is not feasible. Thus, patients who want to participate in choosing treatment will perceive that the information given is adequate to their needs. Others who want the doctor to decide will not have responsibility thrust on them. If the patient perceives the information given as adequate (neither too much nor too little) this will protect against anxiety and depression in the short and long term.

New cancer genetics

With the discovery of BRCA1 and BRCA2, rapid growth has occurred in the demand for information about the risk factors for cancer and advice on risk management from unaffected women with a family history of the disease. A new area of research has been generated, assessing the psychosocial impact of genetic risk communication, genetic testing, and preventive options.

Informing individuals of their personal risk has been shown to improve the accuracy of women's risk perceptions, which are otherwise often estimated to be much lower or higher than the geneticists' risk calculations. This is achieved without any increase in general psychological distress and with a short term reduction in anxiety. Between 20 and 55% of women, however, may fail to correct an inaccurate perception of their risk; this is of concern, because correct risk knowledge is deemed to be the best basis for making decisions about risk management. Results are inconclusive as to whether risk counselling reduces worries about cancer, and as yet too few studies have reported the impact on lifestyle changes or healthcare behaviour.

The impact of preventive breast surgery has attracted considerable research interest, but long term outcomes from prospective studies are awaited. Women who accept preventive surgery have better mental health than those who decline, whereas women who opt for surgery seem to have high levels of satisfaction and report little or no adverse effect on psychological morbidity. Worries about cancer may decline after surgery. Most women opt for bilateral breast reconstruction and the resulting body image seems to be

> **Some women who have breast cancer wish to remain in denial because the reality is too painful to face**

Challenging relatives' wishes to withhold diagnosis from patient

- Explore relatives' reasons but respect them
- Establish potential costs to:
  — Relative
  — Key relationship
- Ask permission to check patient's awareness
- If patient is aware, confirm diagnosis

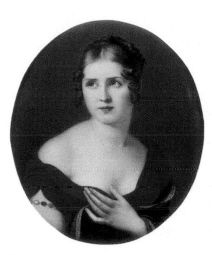

"The Beautiful Greek," Marie Pauline Bonaparte by Counis. Marie Pauline, Napolean's sister, died from breast cancer in 1824. She was 45

> **The psychosocial impact of being a BRCA1 or BRCA2 carrier is being researched, and early findings indicate a transient increase in distress, but also appropriate uptake of surveillance. Women who decline genetic testing or who are found not to be gene carriers may have psychological problems, such as continued anxiety, depression or survivor guilt**

acceptable to most women. Those who develop surgical complications, however, may have psychological and body image problems that warrant further assessment and treatment. Findings are somewhat conflicting with regard to the impact of surgery on sexual functioning, but undergoing bilateral oophorectomy to reduce the risk of ovarian cancer, resulting in an early menopause for younger women, may confound this. Further research is needed to clarify and confirm these important sequelae.

National guidelines for the classification and care of women at risk for familial cancer are helpful to provide a robust framework for future management. The needs for standard information and access to psychological support and advice should be emphasised appropriately in such guidelines.

Support services

These include specialist nurses, volunteers, self help groups, and national organisations.

Specialist nurses

Specialist nurses can check patients' understanding of and reaction to a consultation when bad news is given, and can offer further information and practical and emotional support. Such counselling can reduce anxiety and body image problems but not depression. Appropriately trained nurses can monitor patients' adjustment and recognise most of those who need help and refer them to a psychologist or psychiatrist. This leads to a fourfold reduction in psychological morbidity. Monitoring each patient once within two months of discharge is as effective as regular monitoring. Patients who develop problems later can be relied on to contact the specialist nurse.

Effective training of specialist nurses must ensure that they acquire the skills that promote disclosure and relinquish behaviours that inhibit it. Specialist nurses also need to have regular supervision if they are to remain effective, and they must have rapid access to expert advice from a psychiatrist or clinical psychologist when they uncover severe psychological problems. The use of specialist nurses has disadvantages; other health professionals may leave psychological care to them. Yet it is what treating doctors say about diagnosis and treatment that is critical in determining patients' psychological adaptation.

Focusing on those at risk

Specialist nurses are most effective if they can identify and concentrate on patients who are at risk of affective disorders. Useful markers of risk have been established and include past psychiatric history, low self esteem, perceived lack of support, and having four or more unresolved concerns about their predicament. Self rating scales like the hospital anxiety and depression scale or the Rotterdam symptom checklist can also be used to identify probable cases in a clinic. High scorers then need to be assessed to see if they are true cases of affective disorders and warrant treatment.

Markers of risk for affective disorders

- Past psychiatric illness
- Toxicity as a result of radiotherapy or chemotherapy
- Lymphoedema or pain
- Problems with body image
- No confiding tie
- Low self esteem
- Unresolved concerns

Names and addresses of self help groups

Breast Cancer Care
Kiln House, 210 New Kings Road, London SW6 4NZ
Tel: 020 7384 2984; Fax: 020 7384 3387
email: bcc@breastcancercare.org.uk

Breast Cancer Care (Scotland)
4th floor, 40 St Enoch Square, Glasgow, G1 4DH
Tel: 0845 077 1892
Email: sco@breastcancercare.org.uk
Website: www.breastcancercare.org.uk

CancerBACUP
3 Bath Place, Rivington Street, London EC2A 3JR
Tel: 020 7696 9003
To order CancerBACUP booklets or factsheets
Tel: 020 7696 9003
Website: www.cancerbacup.org.uk

British Association for Counselling and Psychotherapy
Website: www.counselling.co.uk

The Daisy Network (Premature menopause support group)
Email: info@daisynetwork.org.uk
Website: www.daisynetwork.org.uk

Deaf Women Against Breast Cancer
31 Alexandra Drive, Wivenhoe, Chichester, CO7 9SF
Email: deafbc@yahoo.co.uk

Cancer Counselling Trust
Website: www.cctrust.org.uk

Macmillan Cancer Relief
89 Albert Embankment, London SE1 7UQ
Tel: 0845 601 6161 (information line)
Email: cancerline@macmillan.org.uk
Website: www.macmillan.org.uk

Marie Curie Cancer Care
89 Albert Embankment, London SE1 7TP
Tel: 020 7599 7777 (London); 0131 456 3700 (Scotland); 01873 303000 (Wales)
Email: info@mariecurie.org.uk
Website: www.mariecurie.org.uk

Tak Tent Cancer Support—Scotland
Website: www.taktent.org.uk

Volunteers

Patients should be asked if they would like to talk with a volunteer who has been through a similar experience. Appropriately trained volunteers can be contacted through the Breast Cancer Care group. Alternatively, patients may wish to attend a local self help group. Support groups are helpful as long as they are run by people with appropriate experience and sensitivity who are willing to use health professionals as a resource. Advice about coping strategies is particularly helpful.

Support for the family

It is important to check how a patient's partner and other family members are coping. Many relatives believe that they must not compete with the patient's need for help even though they have as many concerns. Those with unresolved concerns are at high risk of later anxiety or depression, particularly if they resent the role changes forced upon them by the patient's illness and treatment and feel dissatisfied with the medical information they have been given.

Dealing with interval cancers

The development of breast cancer within three years of a negative screen can provoke concern that cancer was missed by screening. Specialist nurses should make women aware that they can check on previous findings if they wish. If they do not pursue this offer they should be reminded of it within six months. Women who show no interest in previous findings should not have further information thrust on them.

The screening radiologist is well placed to explain any independent review of the mammograms. The radiologist can explain that there was no evidence of cancer or there was a suspicious area that was judged normal but in hindsight the area represented a cancer and was missed. Women should be asked if they wish to see their mammograms and their wishes should be respected.

Training in communication skills

These skills are not innate or usually acquired through experience. Rigorous scientific studies have confirmed that training, which includes cognitive (evidence base), behavioural (practice key communication tasks under safe conditions and receive constructive feedback), and effective components (reflect on attitudes and feelings), is effective in helping health professionals acquire key skills.

Managing recurrence

Some patients are able to put worry about the future to the back of their minds. Other patients are plagued by uncertainty; their fears should be acknowledged, and they should be asked if they want to know more about their disease status and about signs and symptoms that might herald further deterioration. Negotiating follow-up intervals also helps.

Such patients cope well as long as they remain free of key signs and symptoms and have rapid access to the doctor who treats them if signs or symptoms develop.

Doctors should avoid agreeing with a relative to withhold a diagnosis of recurrence from a patient. It increases psychiatric disorder and hinders the resolution of the relative's grief. Denial of the gravity of the situation by a patient should be challenged by gently confronting her with inconsistencies ("You say you are better but you are still losing weight") or by checking if there is a "window" in her denial ("Is there ever a time when you think that it may not work out as well as you hope?").

Useful websites

- www.cancerhelp.org.uk
- www.nelh.nhs.uk (United Kingdom Electronic Library for Health)
- www.cancer.gov (National Cancer Institute and National Institute of Health United States)
- www.intelihealth.com (drug and medicines information)
- www.dipex.org (database of individual patient experiences)

Further reading

- Fallowfield LJ, Hall A, Maguire GP, Baum M. Psychological outcomes of different treatment policies in women with early breast cancer outside a clinical trial. *BMJ* 1990;301:575–80.
- Fallowfield L, Jenkins V, Saul J, Duffy A, Eves R. Efficacy of a Cancer Research Communication Skills training model for oncologists: a randomized trial. *Lancet* 2002;359:650–6.
- Greer S, Moorey S, Baruch JD, Watson M, Robertson M, Mason A, et al. Adjuvant psychological therapy for patients with cancer: a prospective randomised trial. *BMJ* 1992;304:675–80.
- Harrison J, Maguire P. Predictors of psychiatric morbidity in cancer patients. *Br J Psychiatry* 1994;165:5933–8.
- Harrison J, Maguire P, Ibbotson T, MacLeod R, Hopwood P. Concerns, confiding and psychiatric disorder in newly diagnosed breast cancer patients: a descriptive study. *Psycho-Oncology* 1994;3:173–9.
- Ibbotson T, Maguire P, Selby P, Priestman T, Wallace L. Screening for anxiety and depression in cancer patients: effects of disease and treatment. *Eur J Cancer* 1994;30:37–40.
- Maguire P. Improving the recognition and treatment of affective disorders in cancer patients. In: Granville Grossman K, ed. *Recent advances in clinical psychiatry*. Edinburgh: Churchill Livingstone, 1992:15–30.
- Maguire P, Faulkner A, Booth K, Elliot C, Hillier V. Helping cancer patients disclosing their concerns. *Eur J Cancer* 1996; 32:1486–9.
- Parle M, Jones B, Maguire P. Maladaptive coping and affective disorders in cancer patients. *Psychol Med* 1996;26:735–44.
- Butow P, Lobb EA, Meiser B, Barratt A, Tucker KM, et al. Psychological outcomes and risk perception after genetic testing and counselling in breast cancer: a systematic review. *Med J Aus* 2003;178:77–81.
- Braithewaite D, Emery J, Walter E, Prevost AT, Sutton S. Psychological impact of genetic counselling for familial cancer: a systematic review and meta-analysis. *J Natl Cancer Inst* 2004;96:122–33.
- Contant C, Menke-Pluijmers MB, Seynaeve C, Meijers-Heijboer EJ, Klijn JG, Verhoog LC, et al. Clinical experience of prophylactic mastectomy followed by immediate breast reconstruction in women at hereditary risk of breast cancer (HB(O)C) or a proven BRCA1 and BRCA2 germ-line mutation. *Eur J Surg Oncol* 2002;28:627–32.
- Hatcher MB, Fallowfield L, A'Hern R. The psychosocial impact of bilateral prophylactic mastectomy: prospective study using questionnaires and semistructured interviews. *BMJ* 2001;322:76–9.
- Hopwood P, Lee A, Shenton A, Baildam A, Brain A, Lalloo F, et al. Clinical follow-up after bilateral risk reducing ('prophylactic') mastectomy: mental health and body image outcomes. *Psycho-Oncology* 2000;9:462–72.
- Meiser B, Halliday JL. What is the impact of genetic counselling in women at increased risk of developing hereditary breast cancer? A meta-analytic review. *Soc Sci Med* 2002;54:1463–70.
- van Oostrom I, Meijers-Heijboer EJ, Lodder L, Duivenvoorden HJ, van Gool AR, Seynaeve C, et al. Long-term psychological impact of carrying a BRCA1/2 mutation and prophylactic surgery: a 5-year follow-up study. *J Clin Oncol* 2003;21:3867–74.

P Maguire acknowledges the support of Cancer Research UK. The photograph of the sculpture by Elspeth Bennie is reproduced with permission of David Hayes, director of Landmark Highland Heritage and Adventure Park, Carrbridge, Inverness-shire, where the sculpture is sited. The painting by Counis is reproduced by permission of the Bridgeman Art Library.

16 Carcinoma in situ and patients at high risk of breast cancer

DL Page, NJ Bundred, CM Steel

Two main types of non-invasive (in situ) cancer can be recognised from the histological pattern of disease and cell type. Ductal carcinoma in situ (DCIS) is the most common form of non-invasive carcinoma (making up 3–4% of symptomatic and 20–25% of screen detected cancers). It has increased in frequency because of the widespread use of screening mammography. The increase is across all age groups with a 12% annual increase in women aged 30–39 years and an 18.1% annual increase in women >50 years. Ductal carcinoma in situ is characterised by distortion, distention, and complete involvement by a similar and neoplastic population of cells of adjacent ducts and lobular units. By contrast, lobular carcinoma in situ (LCIS) is rare (<1% of cancers detected by screening) and presents as relatively uniform expansion of the whole lobule by regular cells with regular, round, or oval nuclei. Although each involved lobular unit has a uniform cellular population, the pattern and even cytology may, and often does, vary between units, with some intervening ones being minimally involved or uninvolved. Despite the ease of separating these two processes most of the time, cases with combined features should be regarded as having clinical features of both processes.

Criteria have been agreed to distinguish atypical hyperplasia (with specific histological criteria and validation of clinical implications with follow-up studies) and in situ carcinoma, although heterogeneity of some lesions is best resolved by reporting a lesion as having mixed features, not qualifying for the natural history of DCIS. In general, lesions that involve a few membrane bound spaces only and that measure <2–4 mm in their greatest diameter should be regarded as hyperplastic lesions (with or without atypia) and not in situ carcinoma. Better agreement exists about larger lesions. Even if a patient has greatly enlarged lobular units with partial involvement by foci of atypical ductal hyperplasia, this should not be regarded as DCIS for clinical purposes. The lesions are usually 5–8 mm in size and do not have the natural course of DCIS.

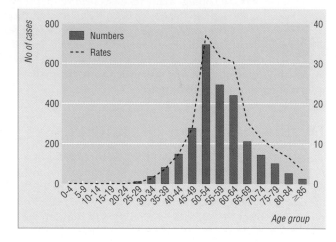

Average number of new cases and rates by age of DCIS 1995–9. Adapted from Cancer Stats, Breast Screening–UK, Cancer Research UK 2003

Classification of DCIS

Histology	Cytology	Necrosis	Calcification
Comedo	High grade	Extensive	Branched
Intermediate	Intermediate	Limited	Limited
Non-comedo*	Low grade	Absent	Microfoci inconsistent

*Cribriform, solid, or micropapillary

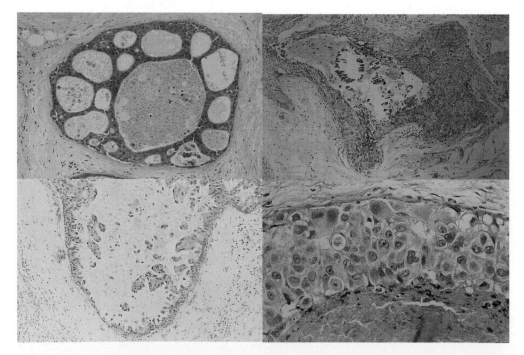

Ductal carcinoma in situ: cribriform DCIS (top left), calcification in an area of DCIS (top right), comedo DCIS (bottom left), and micropapillary DCIS (bottom right). Cribriform and micropapillary, low grade; DCIS with calcification, intermediate grade; comedo DCIS, high grade

Ductal carcinoma in situ

Different classifications of DCIS have been described. Classification based on grade is most widely used. These correlate to some degree with mammographic patterns of microcalcification.

Presentation

Patients with symptomatic DCIS present with a breast mass, nipple discharge, or Paget's disease. Screen detected carcinoma is most often associated with microcalcifications, which may be localised or widespread and characteristically branched within the involved duct system. The microcalcifications are of variable size and density.

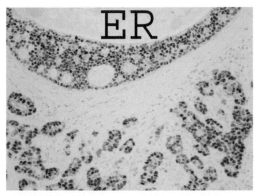

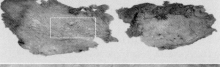

An area of DCIS staining strongly positive for oestrogen receptor

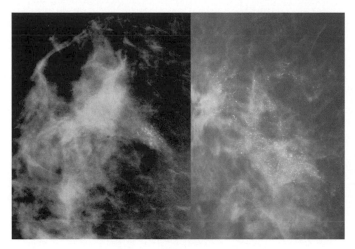

Mammograms showing microcalcification characteristic of DCIS: localised (left) and widespread (right)

Natural course

Several studies have assessed the risk of subsequent invasive carcinoma in patients in whom DCIS was not diagnosed by the pathologist (or the diagnosis was made but mastectomy was not performed). These studies relate to patients with low grade carcinoma in situ, and show that about 40% of them will develop invasive cancer over 30 years, with most of these developing in the first decade. Those who developed invasive cancer did so at the original biopsy site, and they were in the group where the biopsy was thought not to have removed all the DCIS. Information on the behaviour of inadequately excised intermediate and high grade DCIS is derived from therapeutic trials that document local recurrence of DCIS or the development of invasive cancer. The natural course of intermediate and high grade DCIS is continued disease extension and evolution to invasion.

Ductal carcinoma in situ is a heterogeneous group of lesions that differ in growth pattern and cytological features. These lesions have marked biological and behavioural differences. Up to 80% of high grade DCIS overexpresses the oncogene erbB2, whereas only 10% of low grade DCIS expresses erbB2. The presence of a substantial amount of oestrogen receptor also differs between histological grades. Half (range 16–57%) of high grade DCIS are oestrogen receptor positive compared with 70% (range 70–91%) of low and intermediate grade DCIS. Pure cases of micropapillary DCIS, although rare, are usually extensive within the breast and often involve more than a single quadrant.

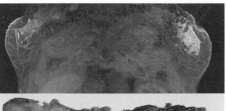

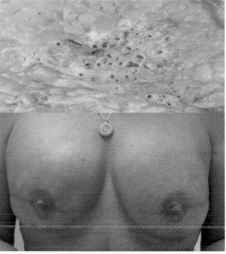

Magnetic resonance image (MRI) scan of a patient (top) with a localized area of nodularity in left breast. No abnormality was seen on mammography or ultrasonography. Core biopsy showed DCIS, and MRI showed a 5 cm area of enhancement that matched the extent of DCIS in the subsequent mastectomy (middle photos). Patient elected to have bilateral mastectomy with immediate reconstruction. Final result after nipple reconstruction and tattooing (bottom)

Treatment

Symptomatic DCIS usually involves much larger areas of the breast than carcinoma in situ detected by screening, and it has traditionally been treated by mastectomy. Such treatment is associated with excellent long term outcome (99% survival at five years). With the advent of breast screening and the use of

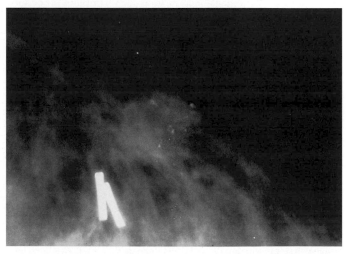

Mammogram of recurrent DCIS seen as microcalcification adjacent to the metal clip in a patient treated by wide excision alone

conservative surgery for invasive carcinoma, wide local excision has been used more often for DCIS. The relative merits of wide excision and mastectomy should be discussed with each individual patient. Ductal carcinoma in situ is increasingly treated by breast conserving surgery with or without postoperative radiotherapy.

Summary of recommended treatment for DCIS*

Localised ductal carcinoma in situ (<4 cm)†
- Wide local excision
- Ensure that mammographic lesion has been completely excised with clear histological margins (at least 1 mm)
- Re-excise if margins are involved
- Consider mastectomy if DCIS >4 cm in size or if micropapillary
- Postoperative radiotherapy (especially if oestrogen receptor or progesterone receptor negative)
- Consider tamoxifen 20 mg a day if oestrogen receptor positive.‡

Widespread ductal carcinoma in situ (>4 cm)†
- Mastectomy (with or without breast reconstruction)
- Tamoxifen not indicated after mastectomy

---

* Outside trials of experimental treatments
† Extent of carcinoma can be estimated in 80% of patients by measuring extent of malignant microcalcification on mammograms
‡ Trails of aromatase inhibitors are under way

Radiotherapy after breast conserving surgery for DCIS
Three randomised trials that involved almost 3000 women have shown about a 50% reduction in the rate of ipsilateral tumour recurrence, but no effect on breast cancer mortality was seen. Disease recurrence is a function of residual disease remaining after initial treatment, because it occurs in the same region and is usually of the same grade as the initial lesion. In the randomised series, not all patients had clear margins. The 1–2% of patients who developed life threatening recurrent disease were distributed equally between the treated and untreated groups. In the European and American trials, an increased risk of contralateral breast cancer was seen after radiotherapy (hazard ratio 2.57 (95% confidence interval 1.24 to 5.33)). High grade DCIS has the highest rate of local recurrence and the greatest benefit from adjuvant radiotherapy. Lesions larger than 4 cm will probably not be excised adequately by wide local excision or quadrantectomy. These lesions seem to have a far higher rate of local recurrence, and so mastectomy is appropriate for extensive areas of DCIS. Axillary surgery is not indicated in localised DCIS; however, axillary node metastases are seen in 1% of high grade lesions larger than 4 cm even when invasion cannot be detected histologically. Patients who have mastectomy for large areas of DCIS should have limited axillary staging by a sentinel node biopsy after a subareolar injection or axillary sampling procedure

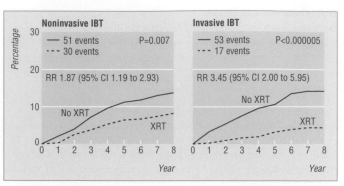

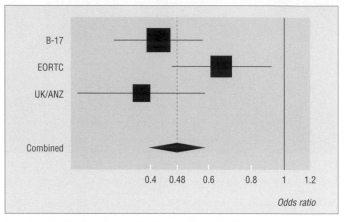

Cumulative incidence of all recurrences of ipsilateral breast tumour and non-invasive and invasive ipsilateral breast tumours and of all other first events in women treated by lumpectomy or lumpectomy and radiation therapy in National Surgical Adjuvant Breast Project Protocol B-17. P values are comparisons of average annual rates of failure. CI = confidence interval; IBT = ipsilateral breast tumour; RR = relative risk; XRT = radiation therapy

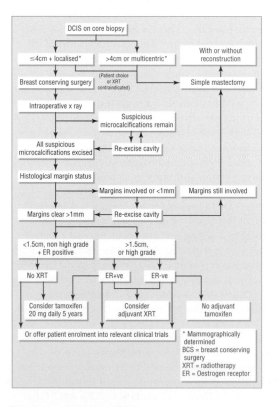

Overview of radiotherapy trials in DCIS: ipsilateral DCIS and invasive recurrences. B-17 = National Surgical Adjuvant Breast Project Protocol B-17, EORTC = European Organisation for Research and Treatment of Cancer, and the UK/ANZ trial is a United Kingdom, Australia and New Zealand study

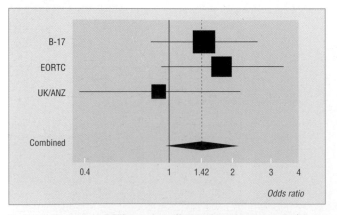

Radiotherapy trials in DCIS overview: all contralateral tumours. B-17 = National Surgical Adjuvant Breast Project Protocol B-17, EORTC = European Organisation for Research and Treatment of Cancer, and the UK/ANZ trial is a United Kingdom, Australia and New Zealand study

Treatment protocol for DCIS

Margin width

Data from three randomised trials have been analysed and margin status and margin width after local excision of DCIS correlated with recurrence. Clear circumferential margins (>1 mm) were associated with a reduction in the risk of recurrence by 30–50% compared with involved margins. Although some have argued that wider margins >1 cm obviate the need for radiotherapy, no randomised trial data exist to support this. Wider margins result in a greater volume excision, which inevitably leads to a poorer cosmetic result.

Factors predicting recurrence after wide local excision of DCIS

Randomised trials have indicated that high grade lesions, comedo necrosis, and incomplete excision of DCIS are associated with a higher rate of local "recurrence." In addition, young age (<50 years) at diagnosis was associated with an increased risk of local recurrence in the American and UK DCIS trials. Local recurrence is in the form of invasive cancer in up to 50% of cases, whereas the remainder of cases are of recurrent DCIS. The European Organisation for Research and Treatment of Cancer study indicated that invasive carcinoma that develops after excision of high grade DCIS is more likely to be node positive than low or intermediate grade invasive "recurrence," regardless of whether radiotherapy is given.

Adjuvant endocrine therapy

Two studies have examined the benefit of tamoxifen in preventing local recurrence. In the American B24 trial, the significant reduction in local recurrence from tamoxifen was predominantly the result of a 40% reduction in women younger than 50 years; older women had a smaller (20%), non-significant reduction. The United Kingdom, Australia, and New Zealand trial found a reduction in recurrent DCIS but not in the development of invasive cancer in patients treated with tamoxifen, but this study included few patients younger than 50 years. A recent pathology review of oestrogen receptor status in a subset of the American trial indicates that tamoxifen reduced the risk of recurrence in oestrogen receptor positive DCIS by 60% (relative ratio 0.41; 95% confidence interval 0.26 to 0.65) but did not affect relapse rate in oestrogen receptor negative DCIS. Thus, there is no indication for using tamoxifen in women with oestrogen receptor negative DCIS or in those who have had mastectomy for DCIS.

Future trials must examine the management of DCIS in specific subgroups (for example, oestrogen receptor positive DCIS) to provide a basis for individualisation of treatment in this condition. One such trial is the International Breast Interventional Study II trial, which compares anastrazole, an aromatase inhibitor, with tamoxifen in women with oestrogen receptor positive DCIS.

Lobular neoplasia (lobular carcinoma in situ or atypical lobular hyperplasia)

Most studies that have reported on this range of lesions have included atypical lobular hyperplasia. Most of these lesions involve separate lobular units and do not show the continuous involvement of adjacent lobular units and ducts that characterise DCIS. No evidence shows that patients with larger lesions or those with more pleomorphic cytology have a higher risk than women with LCIS lesions that are more localised or less pleomorphic.

Presentation

Presentation is often an incidental finding during a breast biopsy, and there are no characteristic clinical or

Risk factors for recurrence of DCIS

Risk factor	Bad prognostic feature	
Excision margins	Margins <1 mm after breast conserving surgery	
Tumour grade	High grade (III)	
Comedo necrosis	Present	
Histological type	Poorly differentiated	
Patient age	Younger age at diagnosis ≤40 years	
Biological markers	*Negativity*	*Positivity*
	Oestrogen receptor	HER2 (erb-B2)
	Progesterone receptor	
	Bcl2	P21
	?erbB4	P53
		Ki67
Patient presentation	Symptomatic	
Tumour size	Not significant	

Recurrence rates for localised DCIS treated by wide excision and radiotherapy in a randomised trial of tamoxifen (National Surgical Adjuvant Breast and Bowel Project B-24)

Cumulative recurrence rate at five years				
Type of recurrence	Cumulative placebo (n = 902)	Tamoxifen (n = 902)	Odds ratio (95% CI)	P value
Ipsilateral noninvasive	5.1	3.9	0.82 (0.53 to 1.28)	0.43
Ipsilateral invasive	4.2	2.1	0.56 (0.32 to 0.95)	0.03
All breast cancer events (includes contralateral disease)	13.4	8.2	0.63 (0.47 to 0.83)	0.0009

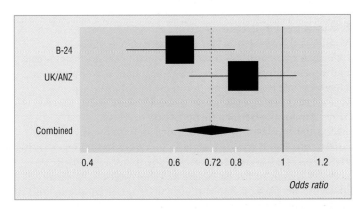

Overview of tamoxifen trials in DCIS. B-24 = National Surgical Adjuvant Breast Project Protocol B-24, and the UK/ANZ trial is a United Kingdom, Australia and New Zealand study

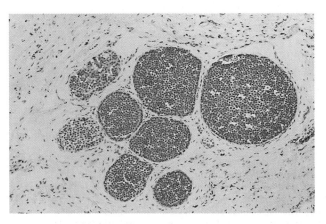

Lobular carcinoma in situ

mammographic features. It is the associated features of dense mammary tissue, enlarged lobular units, and calcifications that are seen on mammograms and explain the increased incidence in the screening population.

Natural course

About 15–20% of women with a diagnosis of LCIS will develop breast cancer in the same breast. A further 10–15% will develop an invasive carcinoma in the contralateral breast.

Treatment

Treatment involves four possible approaches: observation, with yearly bilateral mammography; treatment with a preventative agent; entering the patient into a trial of treatments to prevent breast cancer; or bilateral mastectomy. Bilateral mastectomy should be confined to women who experience severe anxiety that substantially reduces their quality of life. In the National Surgical Adjuvant Breast and Bowel Project tamoxifen breast cancer prevention trial, a 56% reduction was seen in the risk of invasive cancer in patients diagnosed with LCIS who received tamoxifen. Tamoxifen did not, however, reduce the incidence of oestrogen receptor negative or poor prognosis cancers. Ongoing trials are evaluating raloxifene and anastrozole.

Patients at high risk of breast cancer

A variety of risk factors have been identified for breast cancer. Factors that are associated with a slightly elevated risk (<3 times) are not clinically relevant and require no specific action. This includes most of the aspects of lifestyle that are risk factors (age at first pregnancy, history of breast feeding, and diet). The only factors associated with substantially increased risks of subsequent breast cancer are a history of atypical hyperplasia proved by biopsy and family history.

Previous breast disease

Women with palpable breast cysts, particularly women <45 years with multiple cysts, women with certain histological features on biopsy (complex fibroadenomas, duct papillomas, sclerosing adenosis, and moderate or florid usual type hyperplasia) are at a slightly increased risk of breast cancer. Only women with atypical hyperplasia, however, are at substantial (and a clinically relevant) increased risk of breast cancer. Atypical ductal hyperplasia increases in incidence with advancing age but may be associated with a lower relative risk of development of breast cancer in older women. Atypical lobular hyperplasia is less common after the menopause, and it is associated with a lower relative risk when identified in women >55 years. An interaction exists between atypical hyperplasia and family history: women with both atypical hyperplasia and a first degree relative (mother, daughter, or sister) with breast cancer have an absolute risk of 20–30% of developing breast cancer within 15–20 years. Oestrogen replacement therapy given to women with atypical ductal hyperplasia does not produce any greater increase in relative risk than that seen in the general population.

Risk of developing breast cancer associated with risk factors

Factors present	Approximate risk (%)
Atypical hyperplasia (specifically defined)	10–15 in next 15–20 years
Atypical hyperplasia and family history of breast cancer*	20–30 in next 15–20 years
Carrier of mutant BRCA1 gene	55–85 during lifetime
Carrier of mutant BRCA2 gene	37–85
Lifetime risk in general population	12.5

*Disease in first degree relative (mother, sister, or daughter)

Features of ductal carcinoma in situ and localised carcinoma in situ

Feature	DCIS	LCIS
Average age	Late 50s	Late 40s
Menopausal status	70% postmenopausal	70% premenopausal
Clinical signs	Breast mass, Paget's disease, nipple discharge	None
Mammographic signs	Microcalcifications	None
Risk of subsequent carcinoma	30–50% at 10–18 years	25–30% at 15–20 years
Site of subsequent invasive carcinoma		
Same breast	99%	50–60%
Other breast	1%	40–50%

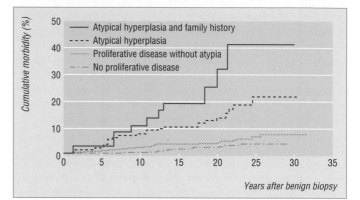

Risk of subsequent development of invasive carcinoma in patients with no epithelial proliferation, proliferative disease without atypia (moderate or florid hyperplasia), atypical hyperplasia, or atypical hyperplasia and a family history of cancer

Relative risk of invasive breast cancer associated with benign diseases

No increased risk
- Mild hyperplasia
- Duct ectasia
- Apocrine metaplasia
- Simple fibroadenomas
- Microcysts
- Periductal mastitis
- Adenosis

Slightly increased risk (1.5–3 times)
- Palpable cysts (cystic disease)
- Moderate and florid hyperplasia
- Papilloma
- Complex fibroadenomas
- Sclerosing adenosis

Moderately increased risk (4–5 times)
- Atypical hyperplasia

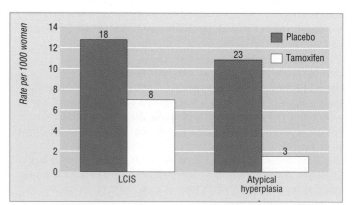

Reduction in invasive breast cancer observed in the National Surgical Adjuvant Breast and Bowel Project tamoxifen breast cancer prevention trial for women with a prior diagnosis of lobular carcinoma in situ (LCIS) and atypical hyperplasia. Diagnosis was based entirely on patient history. Neither the histology report nor the previous histology slides were reviewed

Family history

Up to 10% of patients with breast cancer have a genetic abnormality that predisposes them to develop the disease. The presence of a predisposing breast cancer mutation can be suspected from the following:

- Several cases (strictly speaking, a high proportion) of breast cancer in a single family
- Early onset of breast cancer in affected relatives; not all genetically determined breast cancers present in young women, but the earlier the onset the greater the risk that it is genetic
- Presence of multiple epithelial cancers in family members, including bilateral breast cancer or ovarian, colon, and prostate cancer; the combination of breast and ovarian cancers is particularly common in families with a "cancer gene."

Creating a family pedigree

A family pedigree should be created for people who present with a family history of cancer to confirm that a predisposing mutation is probably present (genetic susceptibility is transmitted as an autosomal dominant trait with limited penetrance) and to estimate the probability that any member of the family has the mutation. The latter is becoming easier to estimate as "breast cancer genes" are identified. At present, however, risk is calculated mainly by statistical methods. Word of mouth histories are often inaccurate or incomplete. To assess risk, it is necessary to extend and verify details of family histories by examining hospital records; pathology reports; data from cancer registers; and public records of births, marriages, and deaths. Now that the BRCA1 and BRCA2 genes have been cloned, it is technically possible to search for mutations in a family with multiple cases of breast cancer. Normally, a blood sample is needed from a living affected family member. The process of screening the whole length of both genes to detect a mutation is laborious and is probably worthwhile in very high risk families only. The same considerations apply to inherited mutations of p53 and PTEN. For members of Ashkenazi Jewish or other genetic groupings where specific BRCA1 or BRCA2 mutations are common, screening may be offered for these mutations for any woman with a positive family history. When a precise causal mutation has been characterised in one affected family member, other at risk relatives can be offered screening.

Genetic testing

Genetic counselling for high risk individuals is critical when genetic testing is an option. Counselling before and after testing is important because of the complexities in the interpretation of test results, management options, and the potential emotional repercussions of test results. From the family history it is possible to assess the likelihood that testing will provide a meaningful result. An important aspect of pretest counselling is an assessment of possible benefits, risks and limitations of genetic testing. Limitations of testing include the possibility that results may not be informative. Even when test results are positive, the risks of a person developing cancer vary from family to family.

Management of women at high risk

Women at high risk of breast cancer may also be at risk of other cancers, and a coordinated approach to their management is

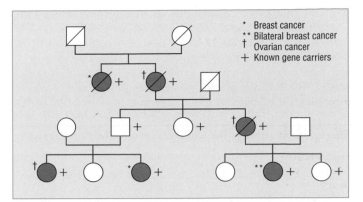

Edinburgh pedigree 2000 with a known BRCA1 mutation. All people who developed breast or ovarian cancer carried a mutated gene. Not all women with the abnormal BRAC1 gene developed breast or ovarian cancer ● = affected members, ○ = unaffected members

> **Carriers of a mutated breast cancer gene may have up to an 80% chance of developing the disease in their lifetime, although some population based surveys put the risk considerably lower**

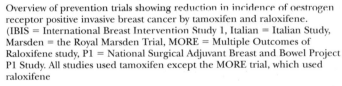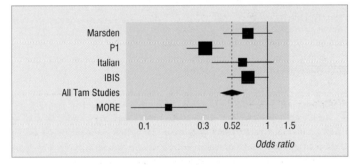

Overview of prevention trials showing reduction in incidence of oestrogen receptor positive invasive breast cancer by tamoxifen and raloxifene. (IBIS = International Breast Intervention Study 1, Italian = Italian Study, Marsden = the Royal Marsden Trial, MORE = Multiple Outcomes of Raloxifene study, P1 = National Surgical Adjuvant Breast and Bowel Project P1 Study. All studies used tamoxifen except the MORE trial, which used raloxifene

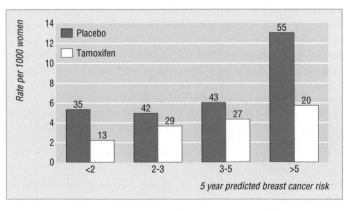

Reduction in invasive breast cancer in the National Surgical Adjuvant Breast and Bowel Project tamoxifen breast cancer prevention trial for groups of women with different relative risks of developing breast cancer

required. Studies have shown that about a third of women with a family history of breast cancer underestimate their own risk by more than half, whereas a quarter of them exaggerate their risk by more than this. Many centres now have clinics for women who have a family history of, or who are at high risk of, breast cancer. These clinics provide genetic counselling and psychological support for these women.

Possible interventions that may reduce mortality in women at risk

- Instituting regular screening
- Preventing development of breast cancer
- Performing bilateral subcutaneous mastectomies

Management strategy for women at increased familial risk*

Family history	Lifetime risk	Risk group	Early mammography†	Refer to genetics clinic
Breast cancer				
One relative <40	1 in 6	Moderate	Yes	No except‡
Two relatives <50 and >40 years	1 in 4–5	Moderate or high	Yes	Yes
Two relatives <60 and >50 years	1 in 5–6	Moderate	Yes	No
Three relatives <60 years	1 in 4	Moderate	Yes	No except‡ and§
One relative with bilateral breast cancer	1 in 3–6	Moderate (unless average age <40 years)	Yes	No except‡ or average age <50 years
Two relatives	1 in 3–4	High	Yes	Yes
Three relatives	1 in 3	High	Yes	Yes
Four relatives	Under 1 in 2 to 1 in 3	High	Yes	Yes
Breast or ovarian cancer				
One ovarian cancer and one breast cancer <50 years	1 in 3–6	Moderate or high	Yes¶ (and ovarian screening)	Yes
More than one ovarian cancer with or without breast cancer at any age	1 in 3	High	Yes¶ (and ovarian screening)	Yes
Childhood cancer				
Childhood tumour	Variable—seek advice	Seek advice	Seek advice (a small proportion will be Li-Fraumeni syndrome)	Yes
<20 years and two other cancers <60 years				

*Table adapted from Sauven P. *Eur J Canc* 2004;40:653–65. The ages in the table are based on average age at diagnosis and the lifetime risks are derived from the Cryllic computer version of the Claus model that gives lower risk than the Claus tables

† Annual mammography from 40–50 years (and then National Health Service Breast Screening Programme (NHSBP))

‡Ethnic origin may make mutation searching and mutation probability higher (for example, in the Ashkenazim who have about a 20% chance of a BRCA1/2 mutation of one of three specific types versus <10% of other Caucasian groups in the United Kingdom)

§Some centres are collecting these families for research for further more moderate risk breast cancer genes

¶Screening for ovarian cancer is not of proven benefit and should be undertaken within a clinical trial only

---

Regular screening

Current recommendations are that women with a strong family history of breast cancer should be screened by mammography, with screening starting at an age five to 10 years younger than that of the youngest relative to have developed the disease. Ultrasonography has been assessed as a screening tool in younger women, but there is no evidence that it is of value. Magnetic resonance imaging (MRI) scans have a higher sensitivity for breast cancer detection than mammography, and current evidence indicates that known BRCA1 and BRCA2 carriers should be screened annually using MRI scans.

Prevention of breast cancer

The National Surgical Adjuvant Breast and Bowel Prevention (NSABP) trial tested the value of tamoxifen as a preventive drug in women whose risk of breast cancer was equal to that of a 60 year old woman. The trial also enrolled patients with atypical hyperplasia, although this information was based on

---

MRI scanning for women at high risk

Three studies (from the United Kingdom, the Netherlands, and Canada) have shown MRI to be a better screening tool than mammography

The UK study (MARIBS study group. *Lancet* 2005;365:1769–78) used 949 women aged 35–49 years with a strong family history or proven genetic mutation. Thirty-five cancers were found by annual screening

- 77% detected by MRI
- 40% detected by mammography
- 94% detected by either MRI or mammography
- Mammography was more specific (93%) than MRI (81%)

Using tamoxifen as a preventative drug in women at high risk is an issue of debate

patient histories and was not validated histologically. After a mean follow up of 47.7 months, there was an 87% reduction in the risk of invasive cancer seen in women considered at risk because of a diagnosis of atypical hyperplasia. The benefits of tamoxifen were seen in all groups of women irrespective of breast cancer risk. No data are available on the group of patients who were gene carriers or those who were at high risk because of family history, but risk reduction was similar in groups of women subdivided by number of relatives affected. The IBIS study confirmed tamoxifen reduced incidence of breast cancer, but there was considerable morbidity associated with its use. Two studies failed to confirm the benefit of tamoxifen. These studies did show that toxicity was generally low for participants on tamoxifen or placebo and that compliance was high. Women who took tamoxifen had an excess of hot flushes, vaginal discharge, and menstrual irregularities. At a median follow up of 4.5 years in the NSABP trial, tamoxifen was found to halve the risk of breast cancer development.

Bilateral subcutaneous mastectomy

Bilateral subcutaneous mastectomy performed five years younger than the youngest family relative to have developed breast cancer might be considered appropriate for women from families that carry BRCA1 or BRCA2 gene mutations as proved by DNA analysis. These operations should be done by experienced surgeons so that as much breast tissue as possible is removed and so that immediate breast reconstruction can be performed. Breast cancers after prophylactic subcutaneous mastectomy, although rare, have tended to occur in the posterior breast, adjacent to the chest wall. This indicates that preservation of the nipple areolar complex with clinical follow up does not reduce the effectiveness of the procedure. Bilateral subcutaneous mastectomy reduces the incidence of breast cancer in women with a family history of breast cancer by about 90%.

Prophylactic oophorectomy

Two large studies have shown that prophylactic oophorectomy can reduce as the risk of subsequent breast cancer by as much as 50%. As BRCA1 and BRCA2 mutation carriers are at increased risk of ovarian cancer prophylactic oophorectomy also reduces the risk of ovarian cancer, although there is small residual risk of primary peritoneal cancer of ovarian type. The fallopian tubes must be removed in the procedure as some "ovarian" cancers in BRCA mutation carriers clearly arise in the tubes.

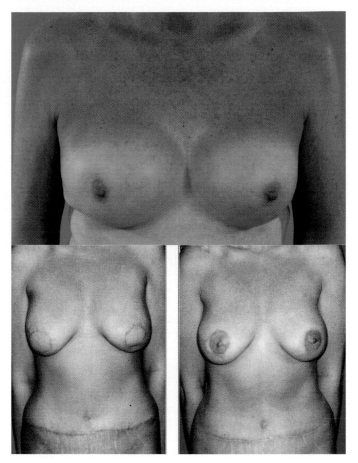

Patient who underwent bilateral subcutaneous mastectomies and immediate breast reconstruction because she was considered to be at high risk of developing breast cancer (top), and patient who underwent bilateral skin sparing mastectomies and immediate free transverse rectus abdominus myocutaneous (TRAM) flap reconstructions with subsequent nipple reconstructions (bottom left and right).

The figure showing average number of new cases and rates of DCIS by age is adapted from Cancer Stats, Cancer Research UK, 2003. The figure showing radiotherapy in DCIS overview for ipsilateral DCIS and invasive recurrences (p 94), and tamoxifen trials (p 95) are adapted from Cruzick J. *J Surg Oncol* 2003;12:213–14.

Further reading

- Burstein HJ, Polyak K, Wong JS, Lester SC, Kaelin CM, et al. Ductal carcinoma in situ of the breast. *N Engl J Med* 2004;350:1430–41.
- Fisher B, Costantino J, Redmond C, Fisher E, Margolese R, Dimitrov N, et al. Lumpectomy compared with lumpectomy and radiation therapy for the treatment of intraductal breast cancer. *New Engl J Med* 1993;328:1581–6.
- Fisher B, Costantino JP, Wickerham DL, Redmond CK, Kavanah M, Cronin WM, et al. Tamoxifen for the prevention of breast cancer: report of the National Surgical Adjuvant Breast and Bowel Project P-1 study. *J Natl Cancer Inst* 1998;90:1371–88.
- Fisher ER, Sass R, Fisher B, Wickerham L, Paik SM. Collaborating NSABP Investigators. Pathologic findings from the National Surgical Adjuvant Breast Project (Protocol 6). I: Intraductal carcinoma (DCIS). *Cancer* 1986;57:197–208.
- Hartmann LC, Sellers TA, Schaid DJ, et al. Prophylactic mastectomy in BRCA1 and BRCA2 mutation carriers. *J Natl Cancer Inst* 2001;93:1633–7.
- Julien J-P, Bijker N, Fentiman IS, Peterse JL, Delledonne V, Rouanet P, et al. on behalf of the EORTIC breast cancer cooperative group and EORT radiotherapy group. Radiotherapy in breast-conserving treatment for ductal carcinoma in situ: first results of the EORTC randomised phase III trial 10853. *Lancet* 2000;355:528–533.
- Kauff N, Satagopan JM, Robson ME, et al. Risk-reducing salpingo-oophorectomy in women with a BRCA1 or BRCA2 mutation. *N Engl J Med* 2002;346:1609–15.
- Page DL. The clinical significance of mammary epithelial hyperplasia. *Breast* 1992;1:3–7.
- Rebbeck TR, Lynch HT, Neuhausen SL, et al. Prophylactic oophorectomy in carriers of BRCA1 and BRCA2 mutations. *N Engl J Med* 2002;346:1616–22.
- Sauven P, on behalf of Association of Breast Surgery Family History Guidelines Panel. Guidelines for the management of women at increased familial risk of breast cancer. *Eur J Cancer* 2004;40:653–65.
- Wolmark N, Digman J, Fisher B. The addition of tamoxifen to lumpectomy and radiotherapy in the treatment of ductal carcinoma in situ (DCIS): preliminary results of NSABP protocol B-24. *Breast Cancer Res Treatment* 1998;50:227.

17 Breast reconstruction

JM Dixon, JD Watson, JRC Sainsbury, EM Weiler-Mithoff

The purpose of the operation is to reconstruct a breast mound to produce breast symmetry. Demand for reconstructive surgery has increased consistently, and up to half of patients offered immediate breast reconstruction choose to have it. No evidence shows that immediate reconstruction increases the rate of local or systemic relapse or that it makes relapse more difficult to detect. Breast reconstruction reduces the psychological trauma experienced by patients after mastectomy. Breast reconstruction (particularly immediate reconstruction, which gives substantially better cosmetic and psychological outcomes) should be more widely available than it is.

Treatment options

The choice of operation for an individual patient depends on several factors. Immediate breast reconstruction is less time consuming for the patient (although not for the surgeon), but care must be taken that the oncological operation is not jeopardised for a better cosmetic result. Reconstruction can be carried out by immediate placement of a prosthesis (implant), but this is rarely practiced. Other options include insertion of a tissue expander or insertion of a flap of skin and muscle (myocutaneous flap) with or without a prosthesis.

Implants and expanders are usually inserted under the muscles of the chest wall (the pectoralis major and parts of the serratus anterior, rectus abdominis, and external oblique); the expander is inflated over several months to stretch the skin and muscle and is eventually replaced with a definitive prosthesis. The two most common myocutaneous flaps used require movement of the latissimus dorsi muscle (with or without overlying skin) or the lower abdominal fat and skin based on the rectus abdominus muscle (transverse rectus abdominus myocutaneous (TRAM) flap). Latissimus dorsi flaps often require a prosthesis to be placed between them and the chest wall to create a breast mound, although by extending the flap to include overlying fat it is often possible to get sufficient bulk without using a prosthesis. Transverse rectus abdominus myocutaneous flaps can be performed as a pedicled flap based

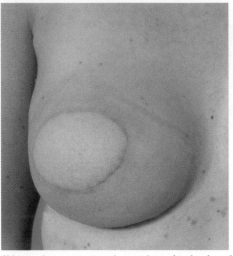

Skin sparing mastectomy in a patient who developed recurrence after breast conserving surgery and radiotherapy (tattooing marks show the area treated). The breast was reconstructed with an extended latissimus dorsi flap with no implant

Options for breast reconstruction

| Technique | Indications for | |
	Immediate reconstruction	Delayed reconstruction
Prosthesis	Small breasts Adequate skin flaps	As for immediate reconstruction *plus* well healed scar *plus* no radiotherapy
Tissue expansion and prosthesis	Adequate skin flaps Good skin closure Small to medium sized breasts	As for immediate reconstruction *plus* well healed scar *plus* no radiotherapy
Myocutaneous flaps	Large skin incision Doubtful skin closure Large breasts	As for immediate reconstruction Can be used if previous radiotherapy

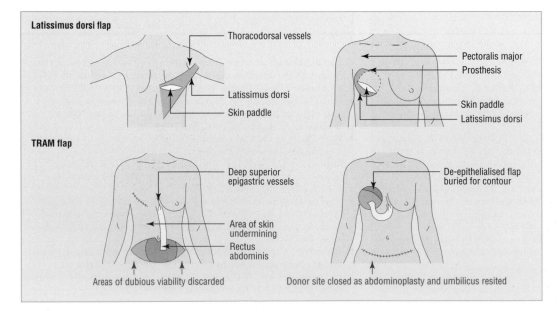

Breast reconstructions with myocutaneous flaps

on the superior epigastric artery or as a free flap based on the inferior epigastric vessels with a microvascular anastomosis. They are bulkier and do not usually need an implant to be inserted. Muscle and fascial harvest may be minimised by raising a perforator flap based on one or two perforators arising from the deep inferior epigastric vessels (DIEP flap). Rates of fat necrosis may be higher during the learning phase with this procedure, as fewer perforators are included in the flap, but the impact on the abdominal wall is less.

All of the above reconstructions can give pleasing results in correctly selected patients when performed by experienced surgeons. All forms of breast reconstruction are substantial surgical operations, and preoperative counseling is essential.

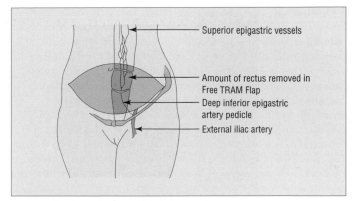

Anatomy of the deep inferior epigastric artery

Tissue expansion and prostheses

The scare about the safety of silicone gel prostheses has put some women off their use. Silicone implants are currently licensed in the United Kingdom and United States for breast reconstructions. The newer silicone implants are "solid" gel implants and come in a variety of shapes and sizes—these are not liquid at body temperature, should have a longer lifespan, and should leak less silicone than liquid silicone implants. Saline prostheses are also available, but they do not have the same doughy consistency of silicone gel and breast tissue. Prostheses can occasionally provide satisfactory results if inserted immediately at the time of operation or as a delayed procedure in patients with small breasts who have adequate skin flaps. Prostheses, however, are generally inserted after a period of tissue expansion. Tissue expansion involves the placement of a silicone bag connected to, or having an integral filler port, with saline injected into the filler port at weekly visits. To achieve ptosis of the reconstructed breast, the expander is inflated to a greater volume than that of the breast mound to be reconstructed before the expander is replaced with a permanent prosthesis. Becker expanders or prostheses that do not need to be removed are available. They consist of two cavities: the outer one containing silicone gel and an inner one that can be inflated with saline. After overinflation, the volume of saline is reduced to obtain the desired volume; the filler port is then removed and the expander or prosthesis is left in situ. Tissue expansion is associated with discomfort of the chest wall and ribs, and the chest wall can be substantially depressed immediately under the expander. Textured tissue expanders seem to produce less chest wall distortion and less discomfort.

It is difficult to create large breast mounds by tissue expansion. If this technique is to be used in a patient with large breasts, the possibility of reducing the contralateral breast should be considered and discussed with the patient.

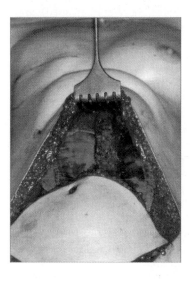

Pedicled TRAM flap being raised for a delayed breast reconstruction

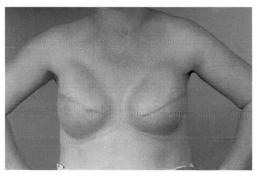

Patient who had immediate placement of bilateral breast prostheses

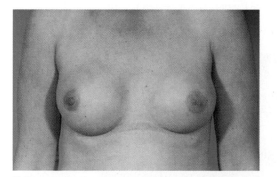

Patient who had a right mastectomy with removal of nipple, but areolar was left intact and left prophylactic mastectomy was reconstructed with bilateral Becker expanders or prostheses. Injection ports can be seen in situ just below and lateral to prostheses

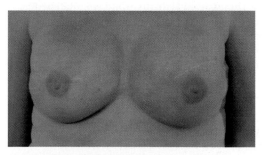

Patient who had bilateral reconstruction with tissue expanders replaced by implants and subsequent nipple reconstructions and tattooing

Radiotherapy

Tissue expansion is difficult in patients who have had chest wall radiotherapy and it is generally not recommended; radiotherapy causes fibrosis in the chest wall muscles and in the overlying skin, which makes it difficult to obtain satisfactory expansion. Such patients are reconstructed better with a myocutaneous flap. Patients who undergo tissue expansion or women with a prosthesis in situ, however, can have postoperative chest wall radiotherapy if this is considered appropriate. This should be delivered over a longer period (in a larger number of fractions) than standard schedules to reduce tissue reaction and fibrosis. One option being explored is to place a temporary subcutaneous prosthesis to retain excess skin. After radiotherapy, the extra retained skin is used as part of a definitive reconstruction. Chemotherapy can be given to patients with prostheses, tissue expanders, or flaps as soon as the wound has healed (areas of skin edge necrosis should preferably have re-epithelialised), and providing there are no signs of underlying infection.

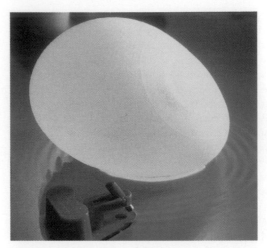

Textured tissue expander used for breast reconstruction having an integral filler part which is located by a magnet as shown

Complications with breast prostheses

Fibrous capsules

The most common complication after the use of prostheses is the formation and subsequent contraction of fibrous capsules around implants. The use of textured prostheses has reduced the incidence of capsular contraction from >50% with smooth implants at one year to <10%. Capsular contraction results in hardening, distortion, an inferior cosmetic appearance of the reconstructed breast mound, and often discomfort and embarrassment. Postoperative or previous radiotherapy substantially increases the rate of capsular contracture. Possible treatments include capsulotomy or capsulectomy, with change of prosthesis to a textured implant if a smooth implant was used. Closed capsulotomy (forced manual rupture of the fibrous capsule) is not an appropriate treatment.

Infection occurs in less than 5% of patients and results in the prosthesis having to be removed. Most units use prophylactic antibiotics to limit the rate of infection. Low grade infection can occasionally manifest as early capsular contraction or erosion of the prosthesis through the overlying skin.

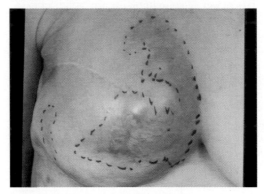

Area of infection over a tissue prosthesis

Implant fatigue and rupture is a major concern among patients, as it leads to leakage of silicone gel. In most patients with ruptured implants, the leakage is intracapsular, with no leakage into the surrounding tissue or body. More than 10% of second generation implants are ruptured or are leaking substantially by 10 years. Ruptured implants seem to cause minimal morbidity as most are intracapsular ruptures. All silicone implants bleed a small amount of silicone gel, although this is much less with the newer generation of low bleed implants. No convincing evidence shows that leaking silicone is carcinogenic or causes problems in other organs. In particular, women with implants do not seem to have a higher rate of connective tissue disorders (such as scleroderma, systemic lupus erythematosus, or rheumatoid arthritis) than age matched women without implants.

The lack of an association between silicone and connective tissue disorders is confirmed by the observation that other patients exposed to silicone (for example, patients with Silicone rubber joints, heart valves containing silicone, or siliconised arteriovenous shunts) do not have an excess of these disorders.

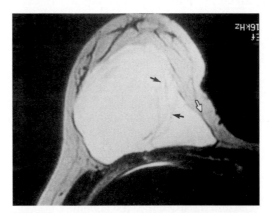

Magnetic resonance image of ruptured implant showing the linguine sign, which represent remnants of the ruptured implant envelope

> Saline filled implants are available for breast reconstruction but have a recognised risk of deflation and produce less satisfactory cosmetic results than silicone filled implants. Soya bean implants are no longer available

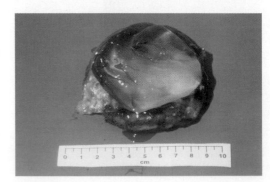

Ruptured implant

Myocutaneous flap reconstructions

These have developed from the early "breast sharing" operations to the recent use of free tissue transfer with microvascular anastomoses. In immediate reconstructions with a myocutaneous flap, skin away from the carcinoma can be preserved (skin sparing), which substantially improves the final cosmetic outcome. Myocutaneous flaps take time and can be performed by one or two teams of surgeons. The emergence of oncoplastic surgeons who perform the cancer operation and the reconstruction has increased the availability of reconstructive surgery.

Latissimus dorsi flaps

First described in 1896 this pedicled flap is a reliable method of breast reconstruction. Although most often used in combination with an implant or a Becker expander or prosthesis, extended flaps that harvest extra fat on the muscle allow purely autologous tissue reconstruction. The thoracodorsal nerve is usually left intact, but it can be divided later if twitching is a problem.

Transverse rectus abdominus myocutaneous flaps

Transverse rectus abdominus myocutaneous flaps can be unipedicled, bipedicled, or free flaps. Free flaps can include muscle, or the surgeon can dissect out the deep inferior perforator vessels as they pass through the muscle leaving the rectus abdominus intact—the DIEP flap. Patients for TRAM or DIEP flaps should ideally be non-smokers and well motivated. Patients who do smoke should cut down on the number of cigarettes they smoke or stop smoking for as long as possible before surgery. Although TRAM or DIEP flaps can be performed on smokers, the incidence of complications associated with smoking is higher. Scarring of the donor site and a prolonged recovery period (up to three months after a TRAM flap) must be discussed fully with the patient. The recovery is shorter after a DIEP flap, because the rectus abdominus is left intact. The use of lower abdominal skin and fat in TRAM or DIEP flaps is often looked on by the patient as a bonus because it gives a cosmetic improvement of the donor site in the form of an abdominoplasty or "tummy tuck".

Complications

Infection can be a problem in latissimus flaps if an implant is inserted. Up to 50% of patients get back wound seromas, but the frequency can be reduced by suturing the skin flaps to the underlying muscle (quilting). The greatest problem with TRAM flaps is necrosis of skin and fat. Major necrosis occurs in up to 10% of patients who have pedicled TRAM flaps, but it affects fewer than 5% of patients with free TRAM flaps. Radiotherapy increases the risk of fat necrosis in TRAM flaps but not extended latissimus flaps. Any fat necrosis is extremely rare after a latissimus dorsi myocutaneous flap, although minor degrees of necrosis can occur in up to 5% of patients. Removal of the rectus abdominis weakens the abdominal wall, and abdominal hernias occur in up to 5% of patients, but they can be reduced by careful abdominal closure.

Nipple reconstruction

In general, it is best to wait at least six months after breast reconstruction before reconstructing the nipple complex to allow the breast time to settle. The nipple complex consists of the nipple and the areola, and each is reconstructed by different methods.

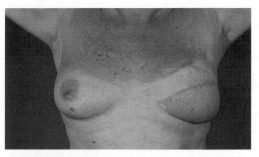

Patient underwent delayed latissimus dorsi flap reconstruction. Because of the high mastectomy scar, the flap was inserted through a separate incision just above the inframammary fold

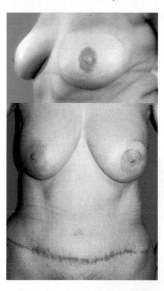

Patient who underwent delayed breast reconstruction with free TRAM flap and nipple reconstruction (top), and patient with an immediate free TRAM flap reconstruction after a skin sparing mastectomy (bottom)

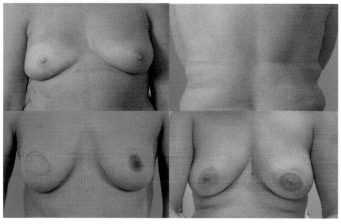

Patient who underwent immediate latissimus dorsi myocutaneous flap reconstruction (top left). Top right shows the back wound. Patient with a skin sparing mastectomy and latissimus dorsi myocutaneous flap (bottom left) and an implant, and patient with a mastectomy and an immediate breast reconstruction with an extended latissimus dorsi flap and later had a nipple reconstruction and nipple tattoo (bottom right)

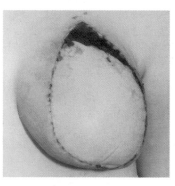

Partial necrosis of upper part of latissimus dorsi myocutaneous flap

Nipple

Several techniques have been devised to make use of local tissue to produce nipple prominence. When the contralateral nipple is particularly prominent, "nipple sharing" is a possibility.

Areola

Dark skin for the new areola used to be obtained from the upper inner thigh, or sometimes part of the contralateral areola was used. Now tattooing is used to recreate the areola, but the colour intensity of the tattooed areola fades with time, so the procedure may have to be repeated.

Use of prosthetic nipples

A false nipple can give a satisfactory shape and colour. An impression is made of the remaining nipple, and a colour matched silicone nipple is prepared by the lost wax technique. This can be prepared in a dental laboratory in two or three days. Patients apply the nipples with medical adhesive and wear them for a month at a time, thereafter peeling them off to wash the skin underneath.

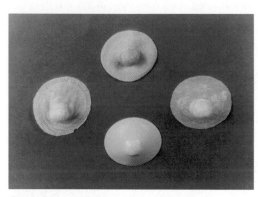

Customised prosthetic nipple (top three) and a commercially available one (bottom centre)

Reduction mammoplasty and mastopexy

It is not always possible to reconstruct a breast mound that matches the natural breast. Both size and shape can pose problems. Major problems with breast reconstructions are that they sit high and proud and often display little ptosis. If a good match of breast volume has been achieved, this lack of ptosis can be hidden by a good bra, thus achieving symmetry when the patient is fully clothed. Some women are happy with this, whereas others want to have the contralateral breast lifted surgically by mastopexy.

When there is a substantial difference in size, symmetry (even when clothed) can sometimes be achieved only by reduction of the natural breast. Some women who have chosen to wear an external prosthesis after a mastectomy and who have no interest in breast reconstruction may also seek reduction of their remaining breast to allow them to wear a smaller and lighter prosthesis.

Complications

These operations can produce considerable permanent scarring, which can be of a variable quality. Delayed skin healing, skin and nipple necrosis, change in or loss of nipple sensation, and an inability to breast feed are specific problems related to reduction mammoplasty and mastopexy.

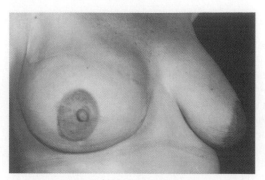

Nipple reconstruction six months after immediate breast reconstruction by a delayed free TRAM flap

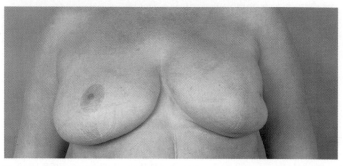

Patient with left breast reconstruction by tissue expansion and prosthesis; she subsequently had her right breast reduced to achieve symmetry

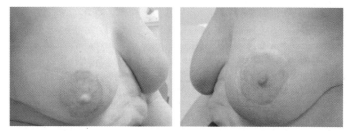

Patient who had a left breast reconstruction with a latissimus dorsi flap and implant and later had a right breast reduction

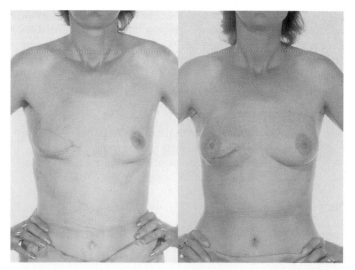

Patient who had right breast reconstruction by latissimus dorsi flap with small implant underneath (left). Subsequently, both the reconstructed and normal breast were enlarged at patient's request and a nipple reconstruction was performed to achieve a better cosmetic result (right)

Other operations

Augmentation mammoplasty after contralateral breast reconstruction

Occasionally, in women with small breasts, the reconstructed side may be larger than their natural breast. This can be corrected by augmenting the unoperated side with a prosthesis filled with silicone gel or saline. Some women take the opportunity of breast reconstruction to achieve larger breasts.

Reconstruction after wide local excision

Tumour size is not a factor associated with local recurrence after breast conservation. The only reason large cancers are treated by mastectomy is that their removal causes a serious volume and cosmetic defect. Options for these large cancers include neoadjuvant therapy, oncoplastic surgery with bilateral simultaneous breast reductions combined with wide cancer excision, or filling the volume defect by means of a local flap such as a latissimus dorsi myocutaneous flap.

This last operation should be done in two stages. Firstly, the cancer is removed and once excision is complete, then a second operation is performed by an axillary incision to remove the axillary lymph nodes and to mobilise the latissimus dorsi muscle and overlying fat so that the breast defect is filled. More than 25% of patients who undergo breast conservation therapy have moderate or poor cosmetic results. To obtain symmetry in these patients, the treated breast usually needs to be augmented in volume by tissue transfer or an implant. If the volume loss is large, transfer of skin and underlying fat or muscle is required. Reduction of the opposite breast may be needed for symmetry.

Revision operations

Patients should have their breast reconstruction performed by a surgeon trained in the whole range of techniques, who can select an appropriate technique of reconstruction for the individual patient. Reconstructive surgery is rarely a single operation, so patients should be warned that to obtain symmetry will require two or three operations. Results should be audited and shown to be of a similar standard to those published in the literature. Some patients, because they develop complications or because of poor symmetry, require major revision of their reconstruction.

Breast cancer after cosmetic breast augmentation

Patients who develop breast cancer after breast augmentation can be treated by breast conserving treatment (wide local excision and breast radiotherapy) if their lesion is appropriate for this approach or by mastectomy. Radiotherapy given to an augmented breast should be delivered over a longer period to reduce tissue reaction and fibrosis around the prosthesis, optimising the final cosmetic result. For women who require a mastectomy, symmetry can be achieved by immediate breast reconstruction.

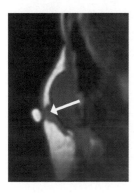

Magnetic resonance image scar of a patient who developed cancer of the breast with an implant in situ. The cancer is arrowed. A palpable lesion was marked by a gel filled capsule on the skin, which is visible on the magnetic resonance image

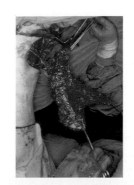

Latissimus dorsi muscle mobilised ready for latissimus dorsi mini-flap reconstruction

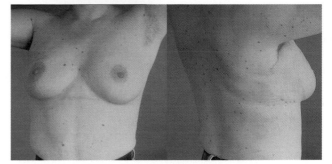

Cosmetic result from mini-flap: front view (left), and side view (right)

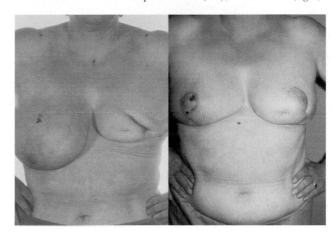

Poor reconstruction result (left) and after revision and reduction (right)

Further reading

- Al-Ghazal SK, Sully L, Fallowfield L, Blamey RW. The psychological impact of immediate rather than delayed breast reconstruction. *Eur J Surg Oncol* 2000;26:17–9.
- Bostwick J, III. *Plastic and reconstructive breast surgery*. St Louis, MO: Quality Medical Publishing, 1990.
- Chawla AK, Kachnic LA, Taghian AG, Niemierko A, Zapton DT, Powell SN. Radiotherapy and breast reconstruction: complications and cosmesis with TRAM versus tissue expander/implant. *Int J Radiat Oncol Biol Phys* 2002;54:520–6.
- Clough KB, O'Donoghue JM, Fitoussi AD, Nos C, Falcou MC. Prospective evaluation of late cosmetic results following breast reconstruction. *Ann Plast Surg* 2001;107:1702–16.
- Cunnick GH, Mokbel K. Skin-sparing mastectomy. *Am J Surg* 2004;188:78–84.
- Gill PS, Hunt JP, Guerra AB, Dellacroce FJ, Sullivan SK, Boraski J, et al. A 10-year retrospective review of 758 DIEP flaps for breast reconstruction. *Plast Reconstr Surg* 2004;113:1153–60.
- Janowsky EC, Kupper LL, Hulka BS. Meta-analysis of the relationship between silicone breast implants and the risk of connective tissue diseases. *N Eng J Med* 2000;342:781–90
- Kronowitz SJ, Robb GL. Breast reconstruction with postmastectomy radiation therapy: current issues. *Plast Reconstr Surg* 2004;114:950–60.
- Shaikh-Naidu N, Preminger BA, Rogers K, Messina P, Gayle LB. Determinants of aesthetic satisfaction following TRAM and implant breast reconstruction. *Ann Plast Surg* 2004;52:465–70.
- Spear SL, Spittler CJ. Breast reconstruction with implants and expanders. *Plast Reconstr Surg* 2001;10:177–87.

Index

Index

Index